FAT BURNING FOODS HANDBOOK

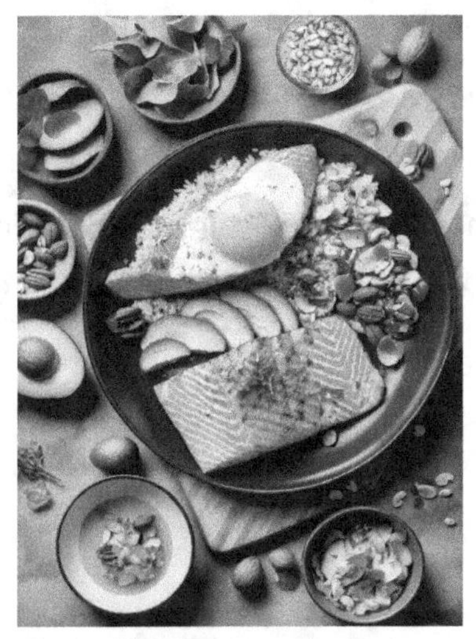

The ultimate fat burning foods handbook for fat and chubby individuals with some frequently asked questions and answers

Dr. Jennifer. V. Albert

1

TABLE OF CONTENTS

Chapter 1:

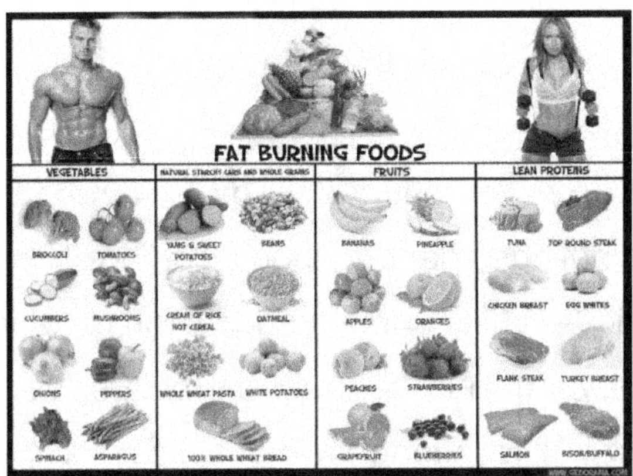

Introduction to Fat–Burning Foods and Metabolism

Introduction to Fat-Burning Foods and Metabolism

Metabolism is a complex biochemical process in which the body converts food and beverages into energy. It's often simplified as the rate at which your body burns calories to sustain life and perform various functions, including breathing, circulating blood, and repairing cells.

Understanding metabolism is crucial for anyone aiming to manage their weight or improve their overall health.

Metabolism is influenced by several factors, including age, gender, body composition, and genetics. While some aspects of metabolism are beyond our control, there are ways to optimize it to support weight loss and overall well-being. One such approach is through the consumption of fat-burning foods.

Fat-burning foods are those that have been shown to increase metabolism or promote fat loss when incorporated into a balanced diet. These foods typically contain specific nutrients, compounds, or properties that enhance metabolic function or stimulate the body's fat-burning processes. While no single food can magically melt away fat, incorporating a variety of these foods into your diet can support your overall weight loss or weight management goals.

One of the key principles behind fat-burning foods is their ability to increase thermogenesis, which is the production of heat in the body. Certain foods have a thermogenic effect, meaning they require more energy to digest, metabolize, and assimilate than other foods. This increased energy expenditure can lead to a higher calorie burn, contributing to weight loss over time.

Additionally, many fat-burning foods are rich in nutrients that support metabolic function. For example, foods high in protein require more energy to digest and can help preserve lean muscle mass, which is essential for maintaining a healthy metabolism. Other nutrients like fiber, vitamins, and minerals play important roles in regulating metabolism, energy production, and fat metabolism.

It's important to note that while fat-burning foods can support weight loss efforts, they are most effective when combined with a balanced diet and regular physical activity. There is no magic bullet for weight loss, and sustainable results are achieved through a holistic approach that includes healthy eating, exercise, adequate sleep, and stress management.

In the following sections, we'll explore the various categories of fat-burning foods, including lean proteins, high-fiber foods, spices and herbs, healthy fats, and more. We'll discuss the specific nutrients and compounds found in these foods that contribute to their fat-burning properties and provide practical tips for incorporating them into your diet. Additionally, we'll explore the role of metabolism in weight management and overall health, dispelling common myths and misconceptions along the way.

By understanding the connection between fat-burning foods and metabolism, you can make informed choices about your diet and lifestyle to support your health and wellness goals. Whether you're looking to shed excess pounds, boost your energy levels, or simply feel better in your body, incorporating fat-burning foods into your routine can be a valuable tool on your journey to better health.

Understanding Metabolism

Understanding Metabolism

Metabolism is a fundamental biological process that encompasses all the chemical reactions occurring within an organism to maintain life. It involves the conversion of nutrients from food into energy that the body uses to carry out various functions, including breathing, circulating blood, regulating body temperature, and repairing cells. Understanding metabolism is crucial for grasping how our bodies function and how they respond to different dietary and lifestyle factors.

Metabolism is often divided into two main categories: catabolism and anabolism. Catabolism refers to the breakdown of larger molecules into smaller ones, releasing energy in the process. This energy is then used to fuel anabolism, which involves the synthesis of larger molecules from smaller ones, requiring energy input. Together, these processes maintain a delicate balance known as metabolic homeostasis, which is essential for overall health and well-being.

The metabolic rate, often simply referred to as metabolism, is the rate at which the body expends energy to carry out its various functions. It is typically measured in calories and can be influenced by several factors, including:

1. Basal Metabolic Rate (BMR): This represents the energy expenditure required to maintain basic bodily functions while at rest, such as breathing, circulating blood, and maintaining body temperature. BMR accounts for the majority of daily energy expenditure and is influenced by factors such as age, gender, body composition, and genetics.

2. Physical Activity: The energy expended during physical activity, including exercise, sports, and daily activities, significantly impacts metabolism. Higher levels of physical activity generally lead to a higher metabolic rate, as more calories are burned to fuel movement and muscle contraction.

3. Thermic Effect of Food (TEF): The energy expended during the digestion, absorption, and metabolism of food is known as the thermic effect of food. Different macronutrients have varying thermic effects, with protein requiring the most energy to digest, followed by carbohydrates and fats.

4. Hormonal Factors: Hormones play a crucial role in regulating metabolism by influencing appetite, energy expenditure, and nutrient storage. Hormones such as insulin, glucagon, leptin, and thyroid hormones are particularly important in this regard.

5. Environmental Factors: External factors such as ambient temperature, altitude, and stress levels can also impact metabolism. For example, exposure to cold temperatures can increase calorie expenditure to maintain body temperature, while chronic stress may disrupt hormonal balance and metabolism.

While some aspects of metabolism are genetically determined, lifestyle factors such as diet, exercise, sleep, and stress management play significant roles in modulating metabolic rate. For example, regular physical activity can increase muscle mass and boost BMR, while a diet rich in whole, nutrient-dense foods can support optimal metabolic function.

Understanding metabolism is essential for effective weight management and overall health. By adopting a holistic approach that includes balanced nutrition, regular physical activity, adequate sleep, and stress management, individuals can support their metabolic health and promote long-term well-being. Additionally, debunking common myths and misconceptions about metabolism can empower individuals to make informed choices about their health and lifestyle. Overall, cultivating a deeper understanding of metabolism can lead to more effective strategies for achieving and maintaining a healthy weight and improving overall quality of life.

How Fat-Burning Foods Work

How Fat-Burning Foods Work

Fat-burning foods are often hailed as a key component of weight loss and metabolic optimization strategies. But how exactly do these foods work to promote fat loss and support a healthy metabolism? Let's delve into the mechanisms behind the effectiveness of fat-burning foods:

1. Thermogenic Effect: Many fat-burning foods have a thermogenic effect, meaning they increase the body's core temperature and metabolic rate. This is often attributed to certain compounds found in these foods, such as capsaicin in chili peppers or catechins in green tea. By raising the body's temperature, these compounds stimulate the metabolism, leading to increased calorie expenditure and potentially enhanced fat oxidation.

2. Increased Satiety: Fat-burning foods are often high in protein, fiber, or both, which can promote feelings of fullness and reduce overall calorie intake. Protein, in particular, has a high satiety value and requires more energy to digest compared to carbohydrates or fats. By including protein-rich foods like lean meats, fish, eggs, and legumes in your diet, you can help control hunger and prevent overeating, ultimately supporting weight loss and fat burning.

3. Regulation of Insulin and Blood Sugar Levels: Certain fat-burning foods, such as whole grains, legumes, and non-starchy vegetables, have a low glycemic index, meaning they cause a gradual rise in blood sugar levels and promote stable insulin levels. By avoiding spikes and crashes in blood sugar and insulin, these foods can help regulate appetite, reduce cravings, and promote fat loss. Additionally, stable blood sugar levels support metabolic health and may reduce the risk of insulin resistance and type 2 diabetes.

4. Promotion of Fat Oxidation: Some fat-burning foods contain compounds that have been shown to enhance the body's ability to burn fat for fuel. For example, medium-chain triglycerides (MCTs) found in coconut oil and certain dairy products have been linked to increased fat oxidation and energy expenditure. Similarly, polyphenols found in foods like green tea, berries, and dark chocolate may stimulate fat breakdown and oxidation, potentially aiding in weight loss and metabolic health.

5. Maintenance of Lean Muscle Mass: Preserving lean muscle mass is crucial for maintaining a healthy metabolism, as muscle tissue burns more calories at rest compared to fat tissue. Fat-burning foods that are rich in high-quality protein, such as chicken, turkey, tofu, and Greek yogurt, can help support muscle growth and repair while promoting fat loss. Including strength training exercises in your fitness routine can further enhance muscle mass and metabolic rate, creating a synergistic effect with fat-burning foods.

6. Modulation of Hormones: Hormones play a significant role in regulating metabolism, appetite, and fat storage. Certain fat-burning foods contain nutrients or bioactive compounds that can influence hormone levels in ways that promote fat loss. For example, omega-3 fatty acids found in fatty fish like salmon and mackerel may improve insulin sensitivity and reduce inflammation, both of which are important for metabolic health and weight management.

In summary, fat-burning foods work through various mechanisms to support weight loss and metabolic optimization. By incorporating a diverse array of nutrient-dense foods into your diet, you can harness the thermogenic, satiating, insulin-regulating, fat-oxidizing, muscle-preserving, and hormone-modulating properties of these foods to achieve your health and fitness goals. However, it's essential to remember that no single food or nutrient can guarantee fat loss on its own. Sustainable weight loss and metabolic health are best achieved through a balanced diet, regular physical activity, adequate sleep, and stress management.

Importance of a Balanced Diet

The Importance of a Balanced Diet

A balanced diet is the cornerstone of good health and well-being. It provides the essential nutrients, energy, and hydration needed for optimal bodily function, growth, and repair. A balanced diet consists of a variety of foods from all the major food groups in appropriate proportions, ensuring that the body receives the right combination of macronutrients (carbohydrates, proteins, and fats), micronutrients (vitamins and minerals), fiber, and water. Let's explore in detail the importance of a balanced diet:

1. Nutrient Adequacy: A balanced diet ensures that the body receives all the essential nutrients it needs to function properly. Each nutrient plays a specific role in maintaining health, from providing energy and supporting growth and development to strengthening the immune system and preventing chronic diseases. By consuming a diverse range of foods, individuals can meet their daily nutrient requirements and optimize their overall health.

2. Energy Balance: A balanced diet provides the right amount of energy to fuel daily activities and support metabolic function. Consuming too many calories can lead to weight gain and obesity, while consuming too few calories can result in malnutrition and fatigue. Balancing energy intake with energy expenditure is essential for maintaining a healthy weight and preventing weight-related health problems.

3. Disease Prevention: A balanced diet rich in fruits, vegetables, whole grains, lean proteins, and healthy fats is associated with a lower risk of chronic diseases such as heart disease, diabetes, cancer, and obesity. These foods are packed with vitamins, minerals, antioxidants, and phytochemicals that have protective effects against inflammation, oxidative stress, and other factors contributing to disease development. By prioritizing nutrient-dense foods, individuals can reduce their risk of developing various health conditions and improve their overall quality of life.

4. Weight Management: A balanced diet is essential for achieving and maintaining a healthy weight. It includes a variety of foods in appropriate portions, helping individuals control their calorie intake while still meeting their nutritional needs. By focusing on nutrient-dense foods that are high in fiber and protein, individuals can feel satisfied and full for longer periods, reducing the likelihood of overeating and promoting weight loss or weight maintenance.

5. Gut Health: A balanced diet that includes plenty of fiber-rich foods supports digestive health and promotes a diverse and healthy gut microbiome. Fiber helps regulate bowel movements, prevents constipation, and feeds beneficial bacteria in the gut, which play a crucial role in immune function, nutrient absorption, and metabolism. Consuming a variety of fruits, vegetables, whole grains, and legumes can help maintain a healthy balance of gut bacteria and reduce the risk of digestive disorders such as irritable bowel syndrome (IBS) and inflammatory bowel disease (IBD).

6. Mental Well-being: Diet plays a significant role in mental health and emotional well-being. Nutrient-rich foods provide the building blocks for neurotransmitters and hormones that regulate mood, stress response, and cognitive function. Research suggests that a diet high in fruits, vegetables, whole grains, lean proteins, and healthy fats is associated with a lower risk of depression, anxiety, and other mental health disorders. By nourishing the body with a balanced diet, individuals can support their mental and emotional health and improve their overall mood and outlook on life.

In conclusion, a balanced diet is essential for overall health and well-being. By prioritizing nutrient-dense foods, maintaining energy balance, and supporting gut health and mental well-being, individuals can optimize their health, prevent chronic diseases, and enhance their quality of life. Embracing a balanced diet as part of a healthy lifestyle can empower individuals to take control of their health and enjoy the numerous benefits of nourishing their bodies with wholesome and nutritious foods.

Chapter 2:

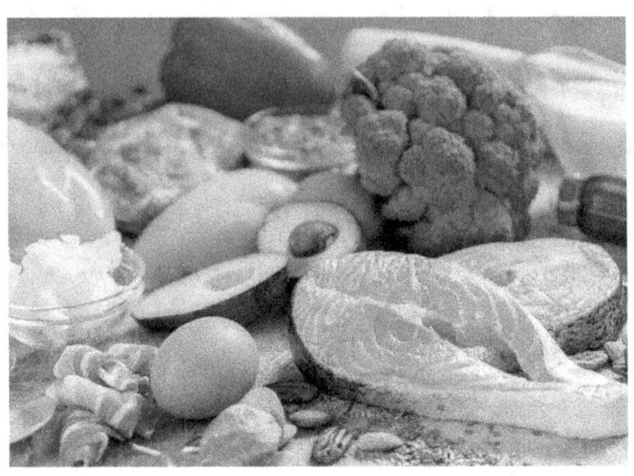

Macronutrients and Their Role in Boosting Metabolism

Macronutrients and Their Role in Boosting Metabolism

Macronutrients are the three main categories of nutrients that provide the body with energy: carbohydrates, proteins, and fats. Each macronutrient serves unique roles in metabolism and can influence metabolic rate in different ways. Understanding how these macronutrients interact with metabolism is crucial for optimizing energy balance, supporting weight management, and promoting overall health. Let's explore the role of each macronutrient in boosting metabolism:

1. Carbohydrates:

- Carbohydrates are the body's primary source of energy and are broken down into glucose, which is used to fuel various physiological processes.

- While carbohydrates have been somewhat demonized in popular diet trends, they play a crucial role in supporting metabolism, particularly during high-intensity exercise and intense physical activity.

- Carbohydrates also stimulate the release of insulin, a hormone that helps transport glucose into cells for energy production. However, excessive consumption of refined carbohydrates and added sugars can lead to insulin resistance and metabolic dysfunction.

- Consuming complex carbohydrates such as whole grains, fruits, vegetables, and legumes provides sustained energy and promotes stable blood sugar levels, which is important for maintaining metabolic health and supporting fat loss.

2. Proteins:

- Proteins are essential for building and repairing tissues, synthesizing hormones and enzymes, and supporting immune function.

- Protein has a higher thermic effect compared to carbohydrates and fats, meaning it requires more energy to digest, metabolize, and assimilate. This increased energy expenditure can boost metabolic rate and promote fat loss.

- Additionally, protein is crucial for preserving lean muscle mass, which is metabolically active tissue that burns calories even at rest.

By consuming an adequate amount of protein, individuals can support muscle growth and maintenance, which can contribute to a higher basal metabolic rate.

- Including protein-rich foods such as lean meats, poultry, fish, eggs, dairy products, tofu, legumes, and nuts in your diet can help increase satiety, control appetite, and promote fat loss while preserving muscle mass.

3. Fats:

- Fats are a concentrated source of energy and play essential roles in cell structure, hormone production, and nutrient absorption.

- Despite their higher calorie content, certain types of fats, such as monounsaturated and polyunsaturated fats found in olive oil, avocados, nuts, seeds, and fatty fish, can actually boost metabolism and promote fat burning.

- These healthy fats support metabolic health by reducing inflammation, improving insulin sensitivity, and enhancing the function of mitochondria, the cellular powerhouses responsible for energy production.

- Including a moderate amount of healthy fats in your diet can help promote feelings of fullness, stabilize blood sugar levels, and support metabolic flexibility, allowing the body to efficiently switch between burning carbohydrates and fats for fuel.

In summary, all three macronutrients—carbohydrates, proteins, and fats—play important roles in metabolism and can influence metabolic rate and fat burning in different ways. A balanced diet that includes a variety of nutrient-dense foods from each macronutrient category is essential for supporting metabolic health, optimizing energy balance, and achieving long-term weight management goals. By focusing on whole, minimally processed foods and paying attention to portion sizes and overall calorie intake, individuals can harness the metabolic benefits of macronutrients to support their health and well-being.

Protein

Protein is one of the three macronutrients essential for human health, alongside carbohydrates and fats. It plays a critical role in numerous physiological processes, including building and repairing tissues, synthesizing hormones and enzymes, supporting immune function, and providing energy. Protein is made up of amino acids, often referred to as the building blocks of protein, which are necessary for the proper functioning of the body.

1. Amino Acids: There are 20 different amino acids that can combine in various ways to form different proteins. These amino acids are classified as either essential or nonessential.

Essential amino acids cannot be produced by the body and must be obtained from the diet, while nonessential amino acids can be synthesized by the body. Consuming a variety of protein sources ensures that the body receives all the essential amino acids it needs for optimal health and function.

2. Sources of Protein: Protein is found in a wide range of foods, including animal-based sources such as meat, poultry, fish, eggs, and dairy products, as well as plant-based sources such as legumes, tofu, tempeh, seitan, nuts, seeds, and certain grains like quinoa and amaranth. Each protein source provides a unique combination of amino acids and other nutrients, making it important to include a variety of protein-rich foods in the diet.

3. Metabolic Role: Protein plays a key role in boosting metabolism and promoting fat loss through several mechanisms:

- Thermic Effect: Protein has a higher thermic effect compared to carbohydrates and fats, meaning it requires more energy to digest, metabolize, and assimilate. This increased energy expenditure can boost metabolic rate and promote fat burning.

- Muscle Preservation: Protein is essential for preserving lean muscle mass, which is metabolically active tissue that burns calories even at rest. By consuming an adequate amount of protein, individuals can support muscle growth and maintenance, which can contribute to a higher basal metabolic rate.

- Satiety and Appetite Control: Protein is the most satiating macronutrient, meaning it helps promote feelings of fullness and satisfaction. Including protein-rich foods in meals and snacks can help control appetite, reduce cravings, and prevent overeating, ultimately supporting weight loss and weight management efforts.

4. Recommended Intake: The recommended dietary allowance (RDA) for protein varies depending on factors such as age, sex, weight, activity level, and overall health status. In general, the RDA for protein is around 0.8 grams per kilogram of body weight per day for adults. However, athletes, older adults, pregnant and breastfeeding women, and individuals with certain medical conditions may require higher amounts of protein to support their unique needs.

5. Quality of Protein: Protein quality refers to the digestibility and bioavailability of the protein in a food source, as well as its amino acid profile. Animal-based sources of protein, such as meat, poultry, fish, eggs, and dairy products, are considered complete proteins because they contain all the essential amino acids in the right proportions. Plant-based sources of protein may be incomplete proteins, meaning they lack one or more essential amino acids, but can be combined to form complete proteins.

6. Protein Timing and Distribution: While the total amount of protein consumed throughout the day is important, the timing and distribution of protein intake may also influence metabolic responses. Research suggests that spreading protein intake evenly throughout the day, with a focus on consuming protein-rich foods at each meal and snack, may optimize muscle protein synthesis, promote satiety, and support metabolic health.

In conclusion, protein is an essential nutrient that plays a critical role in metabolism, muscle function, and overall health. Including a variety of protein-rich foods in the diet can help boost metabolic rate, support fat loss, preserve lean muscle mass, and promote feelings of fullness and satisfaction. By prioritizing protein as part of a balanced diet, individuals can optimize their metabolic health and achieve their health and fitness goals.

Carbohydrates

Carbohydrates are one of the three main macronutrients essential for human health, alongside proteins and fats. They serve as the primary source of energy for the body and play crucial roles in various physiological processes. Carbohydrates are made up of carbon, hydrogen, and oxygen atoms, and they come in several forms, including sugars, starches, and fiber. Understanding the different types of carbohydrates and their impact on health is essential for making informed dietary choices.

1. Types of Carbohydrates:

- Simple Carbohydrates: These are composed of one or two sugar molecules and are quickly digested and absorbed into the bloodstream, leading to rapid spikes in blood sugar levels. Examples include table sugar (sucrose), fruit sugar (fructose), and milk sugar (lactose).

- Complex Carbohydrates: These are composed of long chains of sugar molecules and take longer to digest, resulting in slower and more sustained release of glucose into the bloodstream. Examples include grains (such as wheat, rice, and oats), legumes (such as beans and lentils), and starchy vegetables (such as potatoes and corn).

- Fiber: Fiber is a type of complex carbohydrate that cannot be fully digested by the body. It passes through the digestive tract relatively intact, providing bulk, promoting regular bowel movements, and supporting digestive health. Fiber is found in fruits, vegetables, whole grains, legumes, nuts, and seeds.

2. Metabolic Role:

- Energy Source: Carbohydrates are the body's preferred source of energy, particularly for high-intensity activities and brain function. When consumed, carbohydrates are broken down into glucose, which is used to fuel various physiological processes, including muscle contraction, nerve transmission, and cellular metabolism.

- Glycogen Storage: Excess glucose not immediately used for energy is stored in the liver and muscles as glycogen for later use. Glycogen serves as a readily available source of energy during periods of fasting or increased energy demand, such as exercise.

- Regulation of Blood Sugar: Carbohydrates play a crucial role in regulating blood sugar levels. After a meal, carbohydrates are broken down into glucose, causing blood sugar levels to rise. In response, the pancreas releases insulin, a hormone that helps transport glucose from the bloodstream into cells for energy production or storage.

3. Health Implications:

- Nutrient Density: Carbohydrate-containing foods vary widely in nutrient density. While whole, minimally processed carbohydrates like fruits, vegetables, whole grains, and legumes provide essential nutrients, vitamins, minerals, and fiber, refined carbohydrates like sugary snacks, sweets, and white bread offer little nutritional value and can contribute to weight gain and chronic diseases.

- Blood Sugar Management: Consuming a balanced mix of carbohydrates, proteins, and fats can help regulate blood sugar levels and prevent spikes and crashes in energy. Including fiber-rich carbohydrates in meals and snacks can slow down the absorption of glucose, promote satiety, and support stable blood sugar levels.

- Weight Management: Carbohydrates can play a role in weight management, particularly when consumed in appropriate portions and as part of a balanced diet. High-fiber carbohydrates are more filling and can help control appetite, reduce calorie intake, and promote weight loss or weight maintenance.

4. Recommended Intake:

- The Dietary Guidelines for Americans recommend that carbohydrates make up 45% to 65% of total daily calorie intake for adults. However, individual carbohydrate needs may vary depending on factors such as age, sex, weight, activity level, and overall health status.

- Choosing nutrient-dense carbohydrates from whole, minimally processed sources and limiting intake of refined carbohydrates and added sugars is recommended for promoting overall health and well-being.

In summary, carbohydrates are a vital macronutrient that provides the body with energy and supports various physiological functions. Including a variety of carbohydrates in the diet, particularly from whole, minimally processed sources, can help promote overall health, regulate blood sugar levels, support weight management, and optimize energy levels. By understanding the different types of carbohydrates and making informed dietary choices, individuals can harness the benefits of carbohydrates while minimizing potential health risks.

Fats

Fats are an essential macronutrient that plays numerous critical roles in the body, ranging from providing energy to supporting cell structure and hormone production. While fats have long been demonized in popular culture, they are necessary for optimal health when consumed in appropriate amounts and from the right sources. Let's explore the various aspects of fats in detail:

1. Types of Fats:

- Saturated Fats: Saturated fats are typically solid at room temperature and are found primarily in animal-based foods such as meat, poultry, dairy products, and eggs. They have been associated with an increased risk of heart disease and other health problems when consumed in excess.

- Monounsaturated Fats: Monounsaturated fats are liquid at room temperature and are found in foods such as olive oil, avocados, nuts, and seeds. They are considered heart-healthy fats and have been shown to improve cholesterol levels, reduce inflammation, and lower the risk of cardiovascular disease.

- Polyunsaturated Fats: Polyunsaturated fats are also liquid at room temperature and include two main types: omega-3 and omega-6 fatty acids. Omega-3 fatty acids are found in fatty fish (such as salmon, mackerel, and sardines), flaxseeds, chia seeds, and walnuts, and are known for their anti-inflammatory properties and cardiovascular benefits. Omega-6 fatty acids are found in vegetable oils (such as soybean, corn, and sunflower oil) and nuts and seeds, and while essential for health, they should be consumed in balance with omega-3 fatty acids to maintain optimal health.

- Trans Fats: Trans fats are artificial fats created through hydrogenation, a process that converts liquid vegetable oils into solid fats. Trans fats are found in processed foods such as margarine, fried foods, baked goods, and snack foods and are known to increase LDL cholesterol levels and raise the risk of heart disease. Most health authorities recommend minimizing or avoiding trans fats altogether.

2. Metabolic Role:

- Energy Storage: Fats are the most concentrated source of energy, providing nine calories per gram, compared to four calories per gram for carbohydrates and proteins. Excess energy from food is stored in the body as fat tissue, which serves as a reserve of fuel to be used during periods of fasting or energy deficit.

- Cell Structure: Fats are a vital component of cell membranes, providing structure and stability to cells and facilitating communication between cells. Certain fats, such as omega-3 fatty acids, are particularly important for brain health and cognitive function.

- Hormone Production: Fats are necessary for the synthesis of hormones, including steroid hormones such as testosterone, estrogen, and cortisol. These hormones play crucial roles in regulating metabolism, reproductive function, stress response, and other physiological processes.

3. Health Implications:

- Heart Health: The type and amount of fat consumed can significantly impact heart health. While excessive intake of saturated and trans fats is associated with an increased risk of heart disease, replacing these fats with unsaturated fats can improve cholesterol levels, reduce inflammation, and lower the risk of cardiovascular disease.

- Brain Health: Fats, particularly omega-3 fatty acids, are essential for brain health and cognitive function. Adequate intake of omega-3 fatty acids has been linked to improved memory, mood regulation, and reduced risk of neurodegenerative diseases such as Alzheimer's disease.

- Inflammation: Certain fats, particularly omega-6 fatty acids in excess, can promote inflammation in the body, which is linked to various chronic diseases such as heart disease, diabetes, and arthritis. Maintaining a balanced ratio of omega-3 to omega-6 fatty acids is important for minimizing inflammation and supporting overall health.

4. Recommended Intake:

- The Dietary Guidelines for Americans recommend that fats make up 20% to 35% of total daily calorie intake for adults. However, it's important to focus on consuming healthy fats from sources such as fatty fish, nuts, seeds, avocados, and olive oil, while limiting intake of saturated and trans fats found in processed and fried foods.

- Aim to include a variety of fats in your diet to ensure adequate intake of essential fatty acids and to reap the health benefits associated with different types of fats.

In summary, fats are a crucial macronutrient that plays diverse roles in the body, including providing energy, supporting cell structure, and regulating hormone production. Including a variety of healthy fats in the diet, while minimizing intake of saturated and trans fats, is essential for promoting heart health, brain function, and overall well-being. By understanding the different types of fats and making informed dietary choices, individuals can optimize their fat intake and support their health and longevity.

Chapter 3:

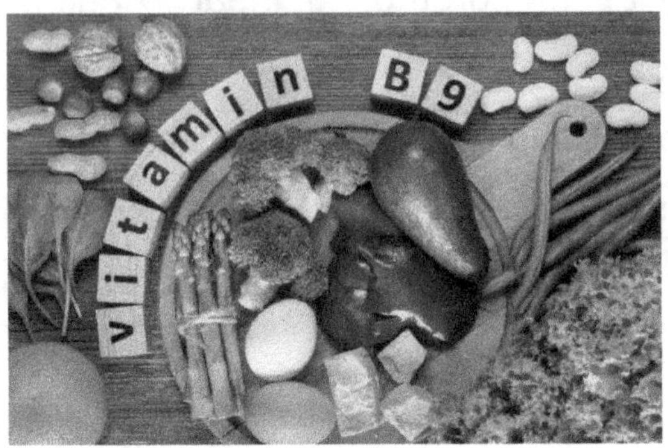

Key Nutrients for
Enhancing Metabolism

Key Nutrients for Enhancing Metabolism

Optimizing metabolism is crucial for maintaining a healthy weight, promoting energy balance, and supporting overall well-being. While various factors influence metabolism, including genetics, age, and physical activity level, certain nutrients play essential roles in metabolic function and energy production. Let's explore some of the key nutrients that can enhance metabolism:

1. Vitamin B Complex:

- The B vitamins, including B1 (thiamine), B2 (riboflavin), B3 (niacin), B5 (pantothenic acid), B6 (pyridoxine), B7 (biotin), B9 (folate), and B12 (cobalamin), are essential for energy metabolism. They act as coenzymes, assisting in the breakdown of carbohydrates, proteins, and fats to produce energy.

- Deficiencies in B vitamins can impair metabolic function and lead to symptoms such as fatigue, weakness, and poor concentration. Including foods rich in B vitamins, such as whole grains, lean meats, poultry, fish, eggs, dairy products, nuts, seeds, legumes, and leafy green vegetables, can help support metabolic health.

2. Vitamin C:

- Vitamin C is an antioxidant that plays a crucial role in energy metabolism and the synthesis of carnitine, a compound involved in the transport of fatty acids into the mitochondria for energy production.

   - Adequate intake of vitamin C is essential for supporting metabolic function, protecting against oxidative stress, and maintaining overall health. Good dietary sources of vitamin C include citrus fruits, strawberries, kiwi, bell peppers, broccoli, and tomatoes.

3. Iron:

   - Iron is a mineral that is essential for the formation of hemoglobin, a protein in red blood cells that carries oxygen from the lungs to the tissues. Iron is also a component of various enzymes involved in energy metabolism and cellular respiration.

   - Iron deficiency can impair oxygen delivery to cells and tissues, leading to fatigue, weakness, and decreased metabolic efficiency. Including iron-rich foods such as lean meats, poultry, fish, tofu, beans, lentils, fortified cereals, and dark leafy green vegetables can help prevent iron deficiency and support metabolic health.

4. Magnesium:

- Magnesium is a mineral that plays a crucial role in over 300 enzymatic reactions in the body, including those involved in energy metabolism, muscle contraction, and protein synthesis.

- Adequate intake of magnesium is essential for supporting metabolic function, regulating blood sugar levels, and maintaining muscle and nerve function. Good dietary sources of magnesium include nuts, seeds, whole grains, legumes, leafy green vegetables, and fortified foods.

5. Zinc:

- Zinc is a trace mineral that serves as a cofactor for numerous enzymes involved in carbohydrate, protein, and fat metabolism. It also plays a role in immune function, wound healing, and DNA synthesis.

- Adequate intake of zinc is important for supporting metabolic health, immune function, and overall well-being. Foods rich in zinc include oysters, red meat, poultry, beans, nuts, seeds, whole grains, and dairy products.

In summary, key nutrients play essential roles in enhancing metabolism and supporting overall health. Including a variety of nutrient-rich foods in the diet, such as fruits, vegetables, whole grains, lean proteins, and healthy fats, can help ensure adequate intake of these important nutrients and support metabolic function. Additionally, maintaining a balanced diet, staying hydrated, getting regular physical activity, and managing stress are important factors for optimizing metabolism and promoting overall well-being.

Vitamin B Complex

Vitamin B complex refers to a group of water-soluble vitamins that play crucial roles in various physiological processes in the body. The B vitamins are essential for energy metabolism, nervous system function, cell growth and division, and the synthesis of hormones and DNA. They act as coenzymes, meaning they assist enzymes in catalyzing biochemical reactions necessary for life. The vitamin B complex consists of eight B vitamins, each with its own unique functions and sources:

1. Thiamine (B1):

- Thiamine is involved in energy metabolism, particularly in the conversion of carbohydrates into energy. It also supports nerve function and plays a role in maintaining a healthy cardiovascular system.

- Good dietary sources of thiamine include whole grains, fortified cereals, pork, nuts, seeds, legumes, and yeast.

2. Riboflavin (B2):

- Riboflavin is essential for energy production, as it is involved in the metabolism of fats, carbohydrates, and proteins. It also plays a role in antioxidant defense and red blood cell formation.

- Dietary sources of riboflavin include dairy products, eggs, lean meats, poultry, fish, fortified cereals, almonds, and leafy green vegetables.

3. Niacin (B3):

- Niacin is important for energy metabolism, DNA repair, and the synthesis of certain hormones. It also helps maintain healthy skin, nerves, and digestive system function.

- Dietary sources of niacin include meat, poultry, fish, peanuts, fortified cereals, whole grains, mushrooms, and leafy green vegetables.

4. Pantothenic Acid (B5):

   - Pantothenic acid is involved in the synthesis of coenzyme A, which is necessary for the metabolism of fats, carbohydrates, and proteins. It also plays a role in hormone synthesis and wound healing.

   - Dietary sources of pantothenic acid include meat, poultry, fish, eggs, dairy products, whole grains, legumes, nuts, and seeds.

5. Pyridoxine (B6):

   - Pyridoxine is involved in over 100 enzymatic reactions in the body, including those related to amino acid metabolism, neurotransmitter synthesis, and hemoglobin formation. It also plays a role in immune function and hormone regulation.

   - Dietary sources of pyridoxine include meat, poultry, fish, potatoes, bananas, chickpeas, fortified cereals, nuts, seeds, and leafy green vegetables.

6. Biotin (B7):

- Biotin is necessary for the metabolism of fats, carbohydrates, and proteins. It also plays a role in gene expression, cell signaling, and maintaining healthy hair, skin, and nails.

- Dietary sources of biotin include egg yolks, liver, nuts, seeds, whole grains, sweet potatoes, and avocado.

7. Folate (B9):

- Folate is essential for DNA synthesis and cell division, making it particularly important during periods of rapid growth and development, such as pregnancy and infancy. It also plays a role in red blood cell formation and amino acid metabolism.

- Dietary sources of folate include leafy green vegetables, citrus fruits, beans, lentils, fortified cereals, and liver.

8. Cobalamin (B12):

- Cobalamin is necessary for red blood cell formation, neurological function, and DNA synthesis. It also plays a role in energy metabolism and the metabolism of fatty acids and amino acids.

- Dietary sources of cobalamin include meat, poultry, fish, shellfish, dairy products, eggs, fortified cereals, and nutritional yeast (for vegans and vegetarians).

In summary, the B vitamins are essential for numerous physiological functions in the body, including energy metabolism, nervous system function, and cell growth and division. Consuming a balanced diet rich in a variety of foods, including lean proteins, whole grains, fruits, vegetables, nuts, and seeds, can help ensure adequate intake of the vitamin B complex and support overall health and well-being. Additionally, certain populations, such as pregnant women, older adults, vegans, and individuals with certain medical conditions, may benefit from supplementation with specific B vitamins to meet their unique needs.

Vitamin C

Vitamin C, also known as ascorbic acid, is a water-soluble vitamin that plays a crucial role in numerous physiological processes in the body. It is a powerful antioxidant that helps protect cells from damage caused by free radicals and oxidative stress. Vitamin C is also essential for collagen synthesis, immune function, wound healing, and the absorption of iron. Let's explore the various aspects of vitamin C in detail:

1. Antioxidant Properties:

- Vitamin C is one of the body's primary antioxidants, meaning it helps neutralize free radicals and reduce oxidative damage to cells and tissues. Free radicals are unstable molecules that can cause cellular damage and contribute to aging, inflammation, and chronic diseases such as cancer, heart disease, and diabetes.

- By scavenging free radicals and preventing oxidative stress, vitamin C helps maintain the integrity of cell membranes, DNA, and proteins, supporting overall health and longevity.

2. Collagen Synthesis:

- Vitamin C plays a critical role in collagen synthesis, the process by which collagen, a structural protein found in connective tissues such as skin, bones, and blood vessels, is produced. Collagen is essential for maintaining the strength, elasticity, and integrity of tissues throughout the body.

- Adequate intake of vitamin C is necessary for healthy skin, hair, and nails, as well as for supporting joint health and preventing conditions such as osteoarthritis and osteoporosis.

3. Immune Function:

- Vitamin C is known for its immune-boosting properties, as it supports the function of various immune cells, including white blood cells and lymphocytes, which help defend the body against infections and diseases.

- Studies have shown that vitamin C supplementation can reduce the severity and duration of colds and respiratory infections, as well as enhance the body's ability to fight off pathogens and recover from illness more quickly.

4. Wound Healing:

- Vitamin C plays a crucial role in wound healing and tissue repair by promoting the production of collagen and other proteins involved in the healing process. It also helps support the formation of new blood vessels, which is necessary for delivering oxygen and nutrients to injured tissues.

- Adequate intake of vitamin C is important for promoting faster wound healing, reducing the risk of infection, and minimizing scarring.

5. Iron Absorption:

- Vitamin C enhances the absorption of non-heme iron, the type of iron found in plant-based foods such as beans, lentils, spinach, and fortified cereals. By forming a complex with iron in the digestive tract, vitamin C helps increase the bioavailability of iron, making it easier for the body to absorb and utilize.

- Consuming vitamin C-rich foods alongside iron-rich foods or iron supplements can help prevent iron deficiency anemia and support overall energy levels and vitality.

6. Dietary Sources:

- Good dietary sources of vitamin C include citrus fruits (such as oranges, lemons, and grapefruits), strawberries, kiwi, guava, papaya, bell peppers, broccoli, Brussels sprouts, kale, spinach, and tomatoes.

- While vitamin C is found in many fruits and vegetables, it is sensitive to heat and light, so cooking and processing can reduce its content. To maximize vitamin C intake, consume raw or lightly cooked fruits and vegetables whenever possible.

In summary, vitamin C is an essential nutrient with a wide range of health benefits. From its antioxidant properties to its role in collagen synthesis, immune function, wound healing, and iron absorption, vitamin C plays numerous critical roles in supporting overall health and well-being. Including a variety of vitamin C-rich foods in the diet, as well as considering supplementation when necessary, can help ensure adequate intake of this important nutrient and promote optimal health throughout life.

Iron

Iron is an essential mineral that plays a crucial role in various physiological processes in the body. It is involved in oxygen transport, energy metabolism, DNA synthesis, and immune function. Iron is also a component of hemoglobin and myoglobin, proteins responsible for carrying oxygen in the blood and muscles, respectively. Let's delve into the diverse aspects of iron:

1. Oxygen Transport:

   - Iron is a key component of hemoglobin, the protein in red blood cells that binds to oxygen in the lungs and carries it to tissues throughout the body. Hemoglobin ensures that cells receive an adequate oxygen supply for energy production and metabolic processes.

   - Iron is also found in myoglobin, a protein in muscle cells that stores oxygen and releases it during periods of increased demand, such as physical activity and exercise.

2. Energy Metabolism:

- Iron is essential for energy metabolism, as it plays a role in the electron transport chain, a series of biochemical reactions that generate adenosine triphosphate (ATP), the body's primary source of energy.

- Iron-containing enzymes, such as cytochromes and iron-sulfur proteins, are involved in various metabolic pathways, including the oxidation of carbohydrates, fats, and proteins to produce energy.

3. DNA Synthesis:

- Iron is necessary for DNA synthesis and cell division, making it essential for growth, development, and tissue repair. Iron-containing enzymes, such as ribonucleotide reductase, are involved in the synthesis of deoxyribonucleotides, the building blocks of DNA.

- Adequate iron intake is particularly important during periods of rapid growth and development, such as infancy, childhood, adolescence, and pregnancy.

4. Immune Function:

- Iron plays a role in immune function, as it is necessary for the proliferation and activity of immune cells, such as lymphocytes and macrophages, which help defend the body against infections and diseases.

- Iron deficiency can impair immune function and increase susceptibility to infections, while adequate iron intake supports a healthy immune response and enhances the body's ability to fight off pathogens.

5. Iron Absorption:

- Iron is obtained from the diet through both heme and non-heme sources. Heme iron is found in animal-based foods such as meat, poultry, and fish and is more easily absorbed by the body compared to non-heme iron, which is found in plant-based foods such as beans, lentils, spinach, and fortified cereals.

- Vitamin C enhances the absorption of non-heme iron by forming a complex with iron in the digestive tract, making it easier for the body to absorb and utilize. Consuming vitamin C-rich foods alongside iron-rich foods or iron supplements can help optimize iron absorption.

6. Iron Deficiency and Anemia:

- Iron deficiency is one of the most common nutrient deficiencies worldwide and can lead to anemia, a condition characterized by low levels of hemoglobin and reduced oxygen-carrying capacity of the blood.

- Symptoms of iron deficiency anemia include fatigue, weakness, pale skin, shortness of breath, dizziness, headache, cold hands and feet, and brittle nails. Severe or prolonged iron deficiency can lead to complications such as impaired cognitive function, delayed growth and development in children, and increased risk of infections.

- Iron deficiency anemia is typically treated with iron supplements and dietary changes to increase iron intake. Including iron-rich foods in the diet, such as lean meats, poultry, fish, beans, lentils, fortified cereals, and leafy green vegetables, can help prevent and alleviate iron deficiency anemia.

In summary, iron is an essential mineral that plays numerous critical roles in the body, including oxygen transport, energy metabolism, DNA synthesis, and immune function. Consuming a balanced diet rich in iron-containing foods, ensuring adequate intake of heme and non-heme iron sources, and considering supplementation when necessary can help support optimal iron status and promote overall health and well-being.

Magnesium

Magnesium is an essential mineral that plays a critical role in numerous physiological processes in the body. It is involved in over 300 enzymatic reactions, making it necessary for energy metabolism, muscle and nerve function, protein synthesis, blood pressure regulation, and bone health. Let's explore the diverse aspects of magnesium in detail:

1. Energy Metabolism:

- Magnesium is a cofactor for several enzymes involved in energy metabolism, including those that facilitate the breakdown of carbohydrates, fats, and proteins to produce ATP, the body's primary source of energy.

- Magnesium helps regulate the activity of ATPase enzymes, which hydrolyze ATP to release energy for cellular processes. It also plays a role in the synthesis of ATP in mitochondria, the energy-producing organelles of cells.

2. Muscle and Nerve Function:

- Magnesium is essential for proper muscle contraction and relaxation, as it regulates calcium ion influx into muscle cells. It helps maintain the balance between excitatory and inhibitory neurotransmitters, which is necessary for normal muscle function and coordination.

- Adequate magnesium intake is important for preventing muscle cramps, spasms, and weakness, as well as supporting nerve conduction and transmission.

3. Bone Health:

- Magnesium is a key component of bone tissue, where it contributes to the formation and maintenance of bone structure. It works synergistically with calcium, phosphorus, and vitamin D to support bone mineralization and density.

- Low magnesium intake has been associated with an increased risk of osteoporosis and bone fractures, as magnesium deficiency can impair bone formation and remodeling.

4. Heart Health:

- Magnesium plays a crucial role in maintaining heart health and cardiovascular function. It helps regulate heart rhythm, blood pressure, and vascular tone, and it supports the relaxation of blood vessels and the prevention of arterial stiffness.

- Adequate magnesium intake has been associated with a reduced risk of hypertension, stroke, and coronary artery disease, while low magnesium levels may increase the risk of heart rhythm disorders and heart failure.

5. Blood Sugar Regulation:

- Magnesium is involved in insulin secretion and glucose metabolism, making it important for blood sugar regulation and the prevention of insulin resistance and type 2 diabetes. Magnesium helps enhance insulin sensitivity and promote glucose uptake into cells.

- Low magnesium levels have been linked to impaired glucose tolerance, insulin resistance, and increased risk of developing type 2 diabetes, while magnesium supplementation may improve glycemic control in individuals with diabetes.

6. Sources of Magnesium:

- Magnesium is found in a variety of foods, including green leafy vegetables (such as spinach, kale, and Swiss chard), nuts and seeds (such as almonds, pumpkin seeds, and sunflower seeds), legumes (such as beans, lentils, and chickpeas), whole grains (such as brown rice, quinoa, and oats), dairy products, fish, and dark chocolate.

- While magnesium is abundant in many plant-based foods, refining and processing can reduce its content. Therefore, consuming whole, minimally processed foods is recommended to maximize magnesium intake.

7. Supplementation:

- In some cases, supplementation may be necessary to meet magnesium needs, particularly for individuals with low dietary intake, malabsorption disorders, or certain medical conditions. Magnesium supplements are available in various forms, including magnesium oxide, magnesium citrate, magnesium glycinate, and magnesium chloride.

- It's important to consult with a healthcare professional before starting magnesium supplementation, as excessive intake of magnesium can cause diarrhea, abdominal discomfort, and other adverse effects in some individuals.

In summary, magnesium is an essential mineral that plays numerous critical roles in the body, including energy metabolism, muscle and nerve function, bone health, heart health, and blood sugar regulation. Consuming a balanced diet rich in magnesium-containing foods, considering supplementation when necessary, and maintaining overall dietary and lifestyle habits that support magnesium status can help promote optimal health and well-being throughout life.

Zinc

Zinc is an essential trace mineral that plays a vital role in numerous physiological processes in the body. It is involved in immune function, protein synthesis, wound healing, DNA synthesis, cell division, and growth and development. Zinc also acts as a cofactor for over 300 enzymes, making it necessary for various biochemical reactions. Let's explore the diverse aspects of zinc in detail:

1. Immune Function:

- Zinc plays a critical role in immune function, as it is necessary for the development and activation of immune cells, including T lymphocytes, B lymphocytes, natural killer cells, and macrophages. Zinc helps regulate immune responses to pathogens and supports the body's defense mechanisms against infections and diseases.

- Adequate zinc intake is important for maintaining a healthy immune system and preventing susceptibility to infections, particularly respiratory infections, gastrointestinal infections, and common colds.

2. Protein Synthesis:

- Zinc is essential for protein synthesis, the process by which cells build and repair proteins necessary for growth, development, and tissue maintenance. Zinc is involved in the transcription and translation of genetic information, as well as in the folding and stabilization of protein structures.

- Zinc deficiency can impair protein synthesis and lead to growth retardation, delayed wound healing, and impaired immune function.

3. Wound Healing:

- Zinc plays a crucial role in wound healing and tissue repair by promoting cell proliferation, migration, and differentiation. It helps regulate the activity of growth factors and cytokines involved in the inflammatory and healing processes.

- Topical application of zinc preparations, such as zinc oxide and zinc sulfate, has been shown to accelerate wound healing and reduce the risk of infection in various skin conditions, including burns, ulcers, and surgical wounds.

4. DNA Synthesis and Cell Division:

- Zinc is necessary for DNA synthesis and cell division, making it essential for growth, development, and reproduction. Zinc-containing enzymes, such as DNA polymerases and RNA polymerases, are involved in the replication and transcription of genetic material.

- Adequate zinc intake is particularly important during periods of rapid growth and development, such as infancy, childhood, adolescence, and pregnancy.

5. Taste and Smell:

- Zinc is involved in the synthesis and secretion of taste and smell receptors, which play a role in detecting and distinguishing various flavors and odors. Zinc deficiency can lead to alterations in taste and smell perception, as well as loss of appetite and decreased food intake.

- Zinc supplementation has been shown to improve taste and smell perception in individuals with zinc deficiency, as well as in elderly individuals with age-related decline in sensory function.

6. Sources of Zinc:

- Good dietary sources of zinc include meat, poultry, fish, shellfish, eggs, dairy products, nuts, seeds, legumes, and whole grains. Animal-based foods, such as red meat and seafood, tend to be higher in zinc compared to plant-based foods.

- While zinc is found in many foods, its bioavailability can be influenced by factors such as food processing, cooking methods, and the presence of phytates and fiber, which can inhibit zinc absorption. Consuming a varied diet that includes a mix of zinc-rich foods can help ensure adequate intake of this important mineral.

7. Supplementation:

- In some cases, supplementation may be necessary to meet zinc needs, particularly for individuals with low dietary intake, malabsorption disorders, or certain medical conditions. Zinc supplements are available in various forms, including zinc gluconate, zinc sulfate, zinc acetate, and zinc picolinate.

- It's important to consult with a healthcare professional before starting zinc supplementation, as excessive intake of zinc can interfere with the absorption of other minerals, such as copper and iron, and may cause adverse effects such as nausea, vomiting, and diarrhea.

In summary, zinc is an essential mineral that plays numerous critical roles in the body, including immune function, protein synthesis, wound healing, DNA synthesis, cell division, and taste and smell perception. Consuming a balanced diet rich in zinc-containing foods, considering supplementation when necessary, and maintaining overall dietary and lifestyle habits that support zinc status can help promote optimal health and well-being throughout life.

Chapter 4:

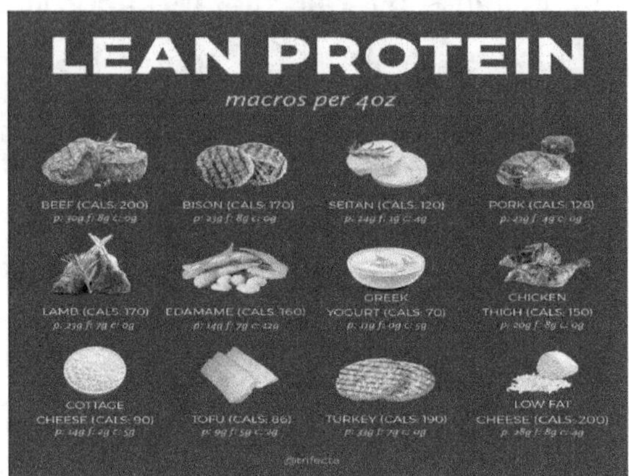

Top Fat-Burning Foods

When it comes to fat burning foods, it's essential to understand that no single food can magically melt away fat. However, incorporating certain foods into your diet can support weight loss and enhance fat burning by boosting metabolism, increasing satiety, and promoting overall health. Here are some top fat-burning foods that you can include in your diet:

1. Lean Protein Sources:

- Lean protein sources such as chicken breast, turkey, fish, tofu, tempeh, legumes, and low-fat dairy products are excellent choices for promoting fat loss. Protein is more thermogenic than carbohydrates or fats, meaning it requires more energy to digest and metabolize, which can boost calorie expenditure.

- Additionally, protein helps preserve lean muscle mass during weight loss, which is crucial for maintaining a high metabolic rate and preventing muscle loss.

2. Whole Grains:

- Whole grains like oats, quinoa, brown rice, barley, and whole wheat contain complex carbohydrates, fiber, and essential nutrients that support fat loss. The fiber content in whole grains helps promote satiety, regulate blood sugar levels, and prevent overeating.

- Consuming whole grains can also help regulate insulin levels, which may aid in reducing body fat storage and promoting fat burning.

3. Fruits and Vegetables:

- Fruits and vegetables are low in calories and high in fiber, vitamins, minerals, and antioxidants, making them excellent choices for weight loss and fat burning. They provide essential nutrients while filling you up with fewer calories, helping to control hunger and reduce overall calorie intake.

- Some fruits and vegetables, such as berries, apples, citrus fruits, leafy greens, cruciferous vegetables, and peppers, are particularly beneficial for fat loss due to their high fiber and water content, as well as their metabolism-boosting properties.

4. Healthy Fats:

- While it may seem counterintuitive, including healthy fats in your diet can actually support fat burning and weight loss. Healthy fats such as avocados, nuts, seeds, olive oil, and fatty fish (like salmon, mackerel, and sardines) provide essential fatty acids and fat-soluble vitamins that are necessary for optimal health and metabolism.

- Additionally, healthy fats help increase satiety, stabilize blood sugar levels, and reduce inflammation, all of which can support weight loss and fat burning.

5. Spices and Herbs:

- Certain spices and herbs have been shown to have metabolism-boosting and fat-burning properties. For example, chili peppers contain capsaicin, a compound that can increase metabolism and promote fat oxidation. Other spices like cinnamon, ginger, turmeric, and black pepper may also have beneficial effects on metabolism and weight loss.

- Adding spices and herbs to your meals not only enhances flavor but can also help rev up your metabolism and support fat burning.

6. Green Tea:

- Green tea is rich in catechins, antioxidants that have been shown to enhance fat oxidation and boost metabolism. Drinking green tea regularly may help increase calorie expenditure and promote fat loss, especially when combined with a healthy diet and regular exercise.

- Additionally, green tea contains caffeine, which can further enhance its fat-burning effects by increasing energy expenditure and promoting thermogenesis.

7. Probiotic-Rich Foods:

- Probiotic-rich foods like yogurt, kefir, kimchi, sauerkraut, and kombucha contain beneficial bacteria that support gut health and may aid in weight loss. Research suggests that the gut microbiota play a role in regulating metabolism and body weight, and consuming probiotic foods may help promote a healthy balance of gut bacteria conducive to fat loss.

- Including probiotic-rich foods in your diet can help improve digestion, reduce inflammation, and support overall metabolic health, all of which contribute to fat burning and weight loss.

It's important to note that while these fat-burning foods can support weight loss and enhance fat metabolism, they should be incorporated into a well-rounded, balanced diet along with regular physical activity for optimal results. Additionally, individual responses to specific foods may vary, so it's essential to listen to your body and find the dietary pattern that works best for you.

Lean Proteins

Lean protein is an essential component of a healthy diet, providing the body with the building blocks it needs for various physiological functions. Unlike protein sources that are high in saturated fats and cholesterol, lean protein sources are low in fat and calories while being rich in essential nutrients. Incorporating lean protein into your diet can support weight management, muscle growth and repair, and overall health. Let's explore lean protein in more detail:

1. Definition and Characteristics:

   - Lean protein refers to protein sources that are low in fat and calories, with a higher protein-to-fat ratio compared to other protein sources. These proteins are typically derived from sources such as poultry, fish, lean cuts of meat, tofu, tempeh, low-fat dairy products, and legumes.

- Lean protein sources provide high-quality protein with minimal added saturated fats and cholesterol, making them ideal choices for individuals looking to maintain or lose weight, support muscle health, and reduce the risk of chronic diseases.

2. Nutritional Composition:

- Lean protein sources are not only rich in protein but also contain essential nutrients such as vitamins, minerals, and amino acids that are necessary for optimal health. They provide essential amino acids, which are the building blocks of protein and play crucial roles in muscle growth, repair, and maintenance.

- Additionally, lean protein sources often contain other nutrients such as iron, zinc, B vitamins, calcium, and omega-3 fatty acids, which support various physiological processes in the body, including metabolism, immune function, and bone health.

3. Benefits of Lean Protein:

- Weight Management: Lean protein is highly satiating, meaning it helps keep you feeling full and satisfied for longer periods, which can aid in reducing overall calorie intake and promoting weight loss or weight maintenance.

- Muscle Health: Protein is essential for building and repairing muscle tissue, especially after exercise or physical activity. Consuming lean protein sources can support muscle recovery, growth, and maintenance, particularly when combined with resistance training or strength exercises.

- Metabolic Health: Protein has a higher thermic effect compared to carbohydrates and fats, meaning it requires more energy to digest, metabolize, and utilize. This increased energy expenditure can support metabolic rate and fat burning, contributing to overall metabolic health.

- Blood Sugar Control: Including lean protein in meals and snacks can help stabilize blood sugar levels and prevent spikes and crashes in energy levels. Protein slows down the digestion and absorption of carbohydrates, resulting in a more gradual release of glucose into the bloodstream.

- Heart Health: Lean protein sources are typically lower in saturated fats and cholesterol compared to fatty cuts of meat and full-fat dairy products. Choosing lean protein options can help reduce the intake of unhealthy fats and lower the risk of cardiovascular disease.

4. Sources of Lean Protein:

- Poultry: Skinless chicken breast, turkey breast, and lean cuts of turkey and chicken.

- Fish: Fatty fish such as salmon, trout, mackerel, and tuna, as well as lean fish like cod, tilapia, and halibut.

- Lean Meat: Lean cuts of beef, pork tenderloin, veal, lamb, and game meats, trimmed of visible fat.

- Plant-Based Proteins: Tofu, tempeh, edamame, seitan, legumes (beans, lentils, chickpeas), and soy products (soy milk, soy yogurt).

- Low-Fat Dairy: Greek yogurt, cottage cheese, skim or low-fat milk, and cheese made from reduced-fat milk.

5. Incorporating Lean Protein Into Your Diet:

- Include a lean protein source in each meal and snack to help meet your daily protein needs and promote satiety.

- Choose a variety of lean protein sources to ensure you get a wide range of essential nutrients.

- Use cooking methods such as grilling, baking, broiling, steaming, and sautéing to prepare lean protein dishes without adding excess fat.

- Be mindful of portion sizes to avoid overconsumption of calories and maintain a balanced diet.

In summary, lean protein is an essential component of a healthy diet, providing the body with high-quality protein and essential nutrients while being low in fat and calories. Including lean protein sources in your meals and snacks can support weight management, muscle health, metabolic function, blood sugar control, and heart health. By incorporating lean protein into your diet, you can optimize your nutrition and promote overall health and well-being.

High-Fiber Foods

High fiber foods are an essential part of a healthy diet, providing numerous health benefits such as improved digestion, weight management, heart health, and blood sugar control. Fiber is a type of carbohydrate found in plant-based foods that the body cannot digest or absorb. Instead, it passes through the digestive tract relatively intact, adding bulk to stools and promoting regular bowel movements. Let's delve into the diverse aspects of high fiber foods:

1. Types of Fiber:

  - There are two main types of dietary fiber: soluble fiber and insoluble fiber.

  - Soluble fiber dissolves in water to form a gel-like substance in the digestive tract. It helps slow down digestion, regulate blood sugar levels, and lower cholesterol levels. Good sources of soluble fiber include oats, barley, beans, lentils, peas, apples, citrus fruits, carrots, and psyllium husk.

- Insoluble fiber does not dissolve in water and adds bulk to stools, promoting regular bowel movements and preventing constipation. It also helps maintain digestive health and prevent diverticulosis. Insoluble fiber is found in whole grains, wheat bran, nuts, seeds, vegetables, and fruit skins.

2. Digestive Health:

- High fiber foods are beneficial for digestive health, as they help regulate bowel movements, prevent constipation, and promote regularity. Fiber adds bulk to stools, softens them, and speeds up transit time through the digestive tract, reducing the risk of constipation and related digestive disorders.

- Additionally, fiber acts as a prebiotic, feeding beneficial bacteria in the gut and promoting a healthy balance of gut microbiota, which is essential for overall digestive health and immune function.

3. Weight Management:

- High fiber foods can aid in weight management by promoting feelings of fullness and satiety, reducing overall calorie intake, and preventing overeating. Fiber-rich foods take longer to chew and digest, which helps control hunger and appetite.

- Furthermore, fiber slows down the absorption of nutrients and sugars in the bloodstream, preventing rapid spikes and crashes in blood sugar levels and promoting stable energy levels throughout the day.

4. Heart Health:

- Fiber is beneficial for heart health, as it helps lower cholesterol levels, regulate blood pressure, and reduce the risk of cardiovascular disease. Soluble fiber binds to cholesterol in the digestive tract and removes it from the body, lowering LDL (bad) cholesterol levels and improving heart health.

   - Additionally, fiber-rich foods like whole grains, fruits, vegetables, legumes, nuts, and seeds are rich in antioxidants, vitamins, and minerals that support heart health and reduce inflammation.

5. Blood Sugar Control:

   - High fiber foods play a crucial role in blood sugar control and diabetes management. Soluble fiber slows down the absorption of sugars in the bloodstream, preventing rapid spikes in blood sugar levels after meals.

   - By promoting more stable blood sugar levels, fiber-rich foods help improve insulin sensitivity, reduce insulin resistance, and lower the risk of type 2 diabetes and metabolic syndrome.

6. Sources of High Fiber Foods:

- Whole Grains: Whole wheat, oats, barley, quinoa, brown rice, bulgur, farro, and whole grain breads and cereals.

- Fruits: Berries (raspberries, strawberries, blueberries), apples, pears, oranges, bananas, kiwi, mango, and avocado.

- Vegetables: Leafy greens (spinach, kale, Swiss chard), broccoli, Brussels sprouts, carrots, sweet potatoes, squash, and peas.

- Legumes: Beans (black beans, kidney beans, chickpeas), lentils, peas, and soybeans.

- Nuts and Seeds: Almonds, walnuts, pistachios, chia seeds, flaxseeds, and pumpkin seeds.

- Other: Psyllium husk, oat bran, and wheat bran.

In summary, high fiber foods are an essential component of a healthy diet and offer numerous health benefits, including improved digestive health, weight management, heart health, and blood sugar control. By including a variety of fiber-rich foods in your meals and snacks, you can optimize your nutrition and promote overall health and well-being. Remember to increase fiber intake gradually, drink plenty of water, and maintain a balanced diet to reap the full benefits of high fiber foods.

Spices and Herbs

Spices and herbs have been used for thousands of years not only to add flavor and aroma to food but also for their medicinal properties and health benefits. From enhancing the taste of dishes to providing therapeutic effects, spices and herbs play a crucial role in culinary traditions around the world. Let's explore the diverse aspects of spices and herbs:

1. Definition and Characteristics:

- Spices are aromatic substances derived from the seeds, bark, roots, fruits, or flowers of plants, whereas herbs are the leaves of plants used for flavoring, culinary, and medicinal purposes.

- Spices and herbs are prized for their distinct flavors, aromas, colors, and textures, which can transform ordinary dishes into culinary delights.

- These flavorful ingredients are often used in dried or ground form, although some are also used fresh or as pastes, extracts, or essential oils.

2. Culinary Uses:

- Spices and herbs are essential ingredients in cooking and baking, adding depth, complexity, and character to a wide range of dishes, including soups, stews, curries, marinades, sauces, salads, and desserts.

- They can be used individually or in combination to create unique flavor profiles and culinary experiences that reflect different cultures and cuisines.

- Common spices include black pepper, cinnamon, cumin, coriander, ginger, cloves, nutmeg, turmeric, and paprika, while popular herbs include basil, thyme, rosemary, parsley, cilantro, mint, oregano, and dill.

3. Health Benefits:

- Spices and herbs are not only flavorful but also packed with beneficial compounds that offer various health benefits. Many spices and herbs possess antioxidant, anti-inflammatory, antimicrobial, and anti-cancer properties.

- For example, turmeric contains curcumin, a potent antioxidant and anti-inflammatory compound that may help reduce inflammation, alleviate pain, and protect against chronic diseases such as heart disease, cancer, and Alzheimer's disease.

- Cinnamon has been shown to help regulate blood sugar levels, improve insulin sensitivity, and reduce the risk of type 2 diabetes, while ginger may aid in digestion, reduce nausea and vomiting, and alleviate muscle pain and soreness.

- Additionally, herbs like basil, thyme, and rosemary are rich in vitamins, minerals, and phytonutrients that support immune function, cardiovascular health, and overall well-being.

4. Medicinal Uses:

- Spices and herbs have been used in traditional medicine systems such as Ayurveda, Traditional Chinese Medicine (TCM), and herbalism for their therapeutic properties and healing effects.

- Certain spices and herbs are believed to possess medicinal properties that can help treat various ailments and conditions, including digestive disorders, respiratory infections, arthritis, headaches, and skin problems.

- For example, garlic is prized for its immune-boosting, antibacterial, and antiviral properties, while peppermint is used to relieve digestive issues such as indigestion, gas, bloating, and irritable bowel syndrome (IBS).

5. Cultural and Culinary Significance:

- Spices and herbs have played a significant role in shaping culinary traditions, cultural identity, and global trade throughout history.

- Many spices and herbs have been highly valued commodities, traded along ancient spice routes that connected distant civilizations and fueled exploration, colonization, and commerce.

- Today, spices and herbs continue to be an integral part of diverse culinary traditions worldwide, reflecting the unique flavors, aromas, and cooking techniques of different cultures and regions.

6. Storage and Usage:

- To preserve the flavor and potency of spices and herbs, it's essential to store them properly in airtight containers away from heat, light, and moisture.

- Spices and herbs should be added to dishes early in the cooking process to allow their flavors to infuse and develop fully. However, delicate herbs like cilantro and parsley are best added at the end of cooking to preserve their fresh flavor and color.

In summary, spices and herbs are versatile ingredients that enhance the taste, aroma, and nutritional value of foods while offering numerous health benefits and medicinal properties. Whether used for culinary purposes, therapeutic applications, or cultural traditions, spices and herbs play an integral role in enriching culinary experiences and promoting health and well-being. Incorporating a variety of spices and herbs into your diet can add excitement and depth to your meals while supporting your overall health and vitality.

Healthy Fats

Healthy fats are essential nutrients that play crucial roles in maintaining overall health and well-being. Contrary to popular belief, not all fats are detrimental to health. In fact, incorporating healthy fats into your diet can provide numerous health benefits, including supporting heart health, brain function, hormone balance, and nutrient absorption. Let's explore the diverse aspects of healthy fats:

1. Types of Healthy Fats:

- **Monounsaturated Fats:** These fats are found in high amounts in foods such as olive oil, avocados, nuts (e.g., almonds, cashews, peanuts), and seeds (e.g., sesame seeds, pumpkin seeds). Monounsaturated fats are known for their heart-healthy benefits, including reducing LDL (bad) cholesterol levels and lowering the risk of heart disease.

- **Polyunsaturated Fats:** These fats include omega-3 and omega-6 fatty acids, which are essential fatty acids that the body cannot produce on its own and must be obtained from the diet. Omega-3 fatty acids are found in fatty fish (e.g., salmon, mackerel, sardines), flaxseeds, chia seeds, walnuts, and hemp seeds. They are known for their anti-inflammatory properties and benefits for heart health, brain function, and joint health. Omega-6 fatty acids are found in vegetable oils (e.g., soybean oil, corn oil, sunflower oil), nuts, and seeds. While omega-6 fatty acids are essential, excessive intake relative to omega-3s may promote inflammation, so it's important to maintain a balanced ratio.

- **Saturated Fats:** While saturated fats have been vilified in the past, emerging research suggests that not all saturated fats are created equal. Certain sources of saturated fats, such as those found in coconut oil and dairy products like yogurt and cheese, may have neutral or even beneficial effects on health when consumed as part of a balanced diet. However, it's still important to consume saturated fats in moderation and prioritize sources of unsaturated fats whenever possible.

2. Health Benefits:

- **Heart Health:** Healthy fats can support heart health by improving cholesterol levels, reducing inflammation, and lowering the risk of heart disease. Monounsaturated fats and omega-3 fatty acids, in particular, have been shown to lower LDL cholesterol levels and triglycerides while increasing HDL (good) cholesterol levels.

- **Brain Function:** Omega-3 fatty acids are essential for brain health and cognitive function. They are important structural components of brain cell membranes and play a role in neurotransmitter function, synaptic plasticity, and neuroprotection. Adequate intake of omega-3s has been associated with improved memory, mood regulation, and reduced risk of neurodegenerative diseases like Alzheimer's disease.

- **Hormone Balance:** Healthy fats are necessary for the production and regulation of hormones, including sex hormones like estrogen, progesterone, and testosterone, as well as hormones involved in appetite regulation, metabolism, and stress response. Consuming sufficient amounts of healthy fats can support hormone balance and reproductive health.

- **Nutrient Absorption:** Fat-soluble vitamins, including vitamins A, D, E, and K, require dietary fat for absorption and utilization in the body. Healthy fats act as carriers for these vitamins, ensuring their proper absorption and distribution to cells and tissues. Incorporating healthy fats into meals can enhance the bioavailability of fat-soluble vitamins and optimize nutrient absorption.

3. Sources of Healthy Fats:

- **Plant-Based Sources:** Olive oil, avocado oil, nuts (e.g., almonds, walnuts, pistachios), seeds (e.g., chia seeds, flaxseeds, hemp seeds), avocado, olives, and coconut (including coconut oil and coconut milk).

- **Fatty Fish:** Salmon, mackerel, sardines, trout, herring, and tuna are rich sources of omega-3 fatty acids, particularly EPA (eicosapentaenoic acid) and DHA (docosahexaenoic acid).

- **Dairy Products:** Greek yogurt, cheese, and milk contain healthy fats, including saturated fats and conjugated linoleic acid (CLA), which may have beneficial effects on health when consumed in moderation.

- **Eggs:** Eggs are a good source of healthy fats, particularly omega-3 fatty acids, when sourced from pasture-raised or omega-3-enriched chickens.

4. Incorporating Healthy Fats Into Your Diet:

- Use healthy oils, such as olive oil, avocado oil, and coconut oil, for cooking and salad dressings.

- Snack on nuts and seeds or add them to salads, yogurt, oatmeal, or smoothies for a nutritious boost.

- Include fatty fish in your diet at least twice a week to increase omega-3 fatty acid intake.

- Enjoy avocados as a spread on toast, sliced in salads, or blended into smoothies for a creamy texture.

- Incorporate whole foods rich in healthy fats, such as olives, coconuts, and eggs, into your meals and snacks.

5. Moderation and Balance:

- While healthy fats offer numerous health benefits, it's important to consume them in moderation and as part of a balanced diet.

- Pay attention to portion sizes and be mindful of total calorie intake, as fats are energy-dense and can contribute to weight gain if consumed excessively.

- Aim to include a variety of healthy fats from different sources in your diet to ensure a diverse range of nutrients and fatty acids.

In summary, healthy fats are essential nutrients that play important roles in supporting overall health and well-being. By incorporating sources of healthy fats into your diet, such as olive oil, avocados, nuts, seeds, fatty fish, and dairy products, you can enjoy their numerous health benefits while enhancing the flavor and nutritional quality of your meals. Remember to consume healthy fats in moderation and as part of a balanced diet to optimize health and vitality.

Green Tea

Green tea is a popular beverage consumed worldwide, known for its refreshing taste and numerous health benefits. Made from the leaves of the Camellia sinensis plant, green tea has been consumed for centuries in traditional Chinese and Japanese cultures and is now enjoyed by people around the globe. Let's delve into the diverse aspects of green tea:

1. Nutritional Composition:

   - Green tea is rich in bioactive compounds, including polyphenols, catechins, and flavonoids, which are potent antioxidants with various health-promoting properties.

   - The most abundant and well-studied catechin in green tea is epigallocatechin gallate (EGCG), which accounts for a significant portion of its antioxidant activity.

- Green tea also contains caffeine, albeit in smaller amounts compared to coffee, as well as amino acids, vitamins (e.g., vitamin C, vitamin K), and minerals (e.g., manganese, potassium).

2. Health Benefits:

- **Antioxidant Properties:** The polyphenols and catechins in green tea act as powerful antioxidants, helping to neutralize free radicals and reduce oxidative stress in the body. This antioxidant activity may help protect cells and tissues from damage and reduce the risk of chronic diseases such as heart disease, cancer, and neurodegenerative disorders.

- **Heart Health:** Green tea has been associated with several cardiovascular benefits, including reducing LDL (bad) cholesterol levels, improving blood vessel function, and lowering blood pressure. Regular consumption of green tea may help lower the risk of heart disease and stroke.

- **Weight Management:** Some studies suggest that green tea may aid in weight loss and weight management by increasing metabolism and promoting fat oxidation. The combination of caffeine and catechins in green tea has been shown to enhance thermogenesis and energy expenditure, leading to greater calorie burning.

- **Brain Health:** The caffeine and amino acids in green tea can improve alertness, focus, and cognitive function. Additionally, the neuroprotective properties of green tea polyphenols may help reduce the risk of age-related cognitive decline and neurodegenerative diseases like Alzheimer's and Parkinson's disease.

- **Blood Sugar Control:** Green tea may help regulate blood sugar levels and improve insulin sensitivity, making it beneficial for individuals with diabetes or at risk of developing type 2 diabetes. The polyphenols in green tea can inhibit carbohydrate digestion and absorption, resulting in lower postprandial blood glucose levels.

- **Immune Support:** The antioxidants and antimicrobial properties of green tea may help strengthen the immune system and protect against infections caused by bacteria, viruses, and fungi. Regular consumption of green tea may reduce the risk of common colds and flu.

3. Varieties of Green Tea:

- There are several varieties of green tea, each with its own unique flavor profile and characteristics. The most popular types of green tea include:

- Sencha: A Japanese green tea with a fresh, grassy flavor and a slightly astringent taste.

- Matcha: A finely ground powdered green tea traditionally used in Japanese tea ceremonies. Matcha has a rich, creamy texture and a slightly sweet, umami flavor.

- Gunpowder: A Chinese green tea characterized by its tightly rolled leaves, resembling pellets or gunpowder. Gunpowder tea has a bold, smoky flavor with a hint of bitterness.

- Dragon Well (Longjing): A renowned Chinese green tea known for its flat, spear-shaped leaves and sweet, nutty flavor. Dragon Well tea is prized for its smooth texture and refreshing taste.

- Gyokuro: A premium Japanese green tea cultivated in the shade to enhance its flavor and aroma. Gyokuro has a sweet, savory taste with a rich, umami finish.

4. Preparation and Consumption:

- To prepare green tea, steep 1-2 teaspoons of loose green tea leaves or a tea bag in hot water (not boiling) for 2-3 minutes for a mild flavor or up to 5 minutes for a stronger brew.

- Green tea can be enjoyed plain or with a slice of lemon, a sprig of mint, or a touch of honey for added flavor. It can be served hot or cold, depending on personal preference.

- It's important not to overbrew green tea or use water that is too hot, as this can result in a bitter taste and astringent mouthfeel.

5. Cautions and Considerations:

- While green tea is generally safe for most people when consumed in moderation, excessive intake may lead to caffeine-related side effects such as insomnia, jitteriness, and heart palpitations.

- Some individuals may be sensitive to the caffeine content in green tea and should limit their intake accordingly, particularly pregnant women, nursing mothers, individuals with anxiety disorders, and those with certain medical conditions.

- Green tea supplements and extracts may contain higher concentrations of catechins and caffeine than brewed tea, so caution should be exercised when using these products.

In summary, green tea is a versatile and health-promoting beverage that offers a wide range of benefits for overall health and well-being. Whether enjoyed for its refreshing taste, antioxidant properties, or potential health benefits, green tea is a popular choice for tea enthusiasts and health-conscious individuals alike. By incorporating green tea into your daily routine, you can reap the numerous benefits of this ancient beverage while savoring its delicious flavor and aroma.

Citrus Fruits

Citrus fruits are a diverse group of fruits belonging to the Rutaceae family, known for their bright colors, refreshing flavors, and numerous health benefits. Native to tropical and subtropical regions, citrus fruits have been cultivated for thousands of years and are enjoyed worldwide for their culinary versatility and nutritional value. Let's explore the diverse aspects of citrus fruits:

1. Varieties of Citrus Fruits:

- Citrus fruits encompass a wide range of species, cultivars, and hybrids, each with its own unique characteristics and flavors. Some of the most common citrus fruits include:

- Oranges: Varieties include navel oranges, Valencia oranges, blood oranges, and mandarin oranges (e.g., tangerines, clementines).

- Lemons: Known for their tart flavor and acidic juice, lemons are commonly used in cooking, baking, and beverages.

- Limes: Limes come in several varieties, including Persian limes (commonly used in culinary applications), Key limes (known for their intense flavor), and kaffir limes (used for their leaves and zest in Southeast Asian cuisine).

- Grapefruits: Available in white, pink, and red varieties, grapefruits are known for their tangy-sweet flavor and juicy flesh.

- Mandarins and Tangerines: These small, easy-to-peel citrus fruits are sweet, juicy, and often seedless, making them popular snacks for both children and adults.

2. Nutritional Composition:

- Citrus fruits are rich in essential nutrients, including vitamin C, folate, potassium, and dietary fiber. They are also low in calories and contain no cholesterol or saturated fats.

- Vitamin C, also known as ascorbic acid, is a powerful antioxidant that plays a critical role in immune function, collagen synthesis, wound healing, and iron absorption. Citrus fruits are one of the best sources of vitamin C, with a single medium-sized orange providing over 100% of the recommended daily intake.

- Folate (vitamin B9) is important for DNA synthesis, cell division, and fetal development during pregnancy. Citrus fruits like oranges and grapefruits are good sources of folate, making them beneficial for pregnant women.

- Potassium is an essential mineral that helps regulate blood pressure, fluid balance, and muscle contractions. Citrus fruits like oranges, grapefruits, and tangerines are naturally rich in potassium and can contribute to a balanced diet.

3. Health Benefits:

- Immune Support: Citrus fruits are renowned for their high vitamin C content, which is essential for a healthy immune system. Regular consumption of citrus fruits may help reduce the duration and severity of colds, flu, and other respiratory infections.

- Heart Health: The antioxidants, flavonoids, and fiber found in citrus fruits have been linked to various cardiovascular benefits, including reducing the risk of heart disease, stroke, and hypertension. Citrus fruits may help lower LDL (bad) cholesterol levels, improve blood vessel function, and decrease inflammation.

- Digestive Health: The dietary fiber found in citrus fruits, particularly in the pulp and peel, promotes digestive health by supporting regular bowel movements, preventing constipation, and feeding beneficial gut bacteria. Citrus fruits can also help maintain a healthy weight by promoting satiety and reducing calorie intake.

- Skin Health: Vitamin C plays a crucial role in collagen synthesis, which is essential for maintaining healthy skin, hair, and nails. The antioxidant properties of citrus fruits may also help protect skin cells from damage caused by UV radiation and environmental pollutants.

- Cancer Prevention: Some studies suggest that the bioactive compounds in citrus fruits, including flavonoids and limonoids, may have anticancer properties and help reduce the risk of certain types of cancer, including breast, prostate, and colon cancer.

4. Culinary Uses:

- Citrus fruits are prized for their versatility in cooking, baking, and beverage preparation. They can be enjoyed fresh, juiced, zested, sliced, or incorporated into a wide range of recipes, from salads and marinades to desserts and cocktails.

- The juice, zest, and pulp of citrus fruits add bright, tangy flavors to both sweet and savory dishes, enhancing their taste and aroma. Lemons and limes are commonly used to add acidity and freshness to salads, sauces, dressings, and marinades, while oranges and grapefruits are popular in desserts, smoothies, and cocktails.

- Citrus fruits can also be candied, preserved, or used to make jams, marmalades, and fruit compotes. The zest of citrus fruits is often used to flavor baked goods, desserts, and savory dishes, while the juice can be used to make refreshing beverages, sorbets, and syrups.

5. Cultivation and Harvest:

- Citrus fruits are typically grown in subtropical and Mediterranean climates, where they thrive in warm temperatures and well-drained soil. Major citrus-producing regions include Spain, the United States (particularly Florida and California), Brazil, China, and India.

- Citrus fruits are harvested when they reach peak ripeness, which varies depending on the variety and growing conditions. Oranges, for example, are typically harvested in the winter months, while lemons and limes may be harvested year-round.

- Citrus fruits are usually handpicked to avoid damaging the delicate skin and bruising the fruit. Once harvested, they are sorted, graded, and transported to markets and distribution centers for sale to consumers.

In summary, citrus fruits are not only delicious but also nutritious, offering a wide range of health benefits and culinary possibilities. Whether enjoyed fresh, juiced, or incorporated into recipes, citrus fruits are a flavorful and refreshing addition to any diet. By including a variety of citrus fruits in your meals and snacks, you can boost your intake of essential nutrients, support your immune system, and promote overall health and well-being.

Berries

Berries are a diverse group of small, colorful fruits that belong to various plant families, each with its own unique flavor, texture, and nutritional profile. From sweet strawberries to tart cranberries, berries are prized for their delicious taste, vibrant colors, and numerous health benefits. Let's explore the diverse aspects of berries:

1. Varieties of Berries:

- Strawberries: These bright red berries are one of the most popular and widely consumed berries worldwide. They have a sweet, juicy flesh and are rich in vitamin C, manganese, and antioxidants such as anthocyanins and ellagic acid.

- Blueberries: Blueberries are renowned for their deep blue-purple color and sweet-tart flavor. They are packed with antioxidants, particularly flavonoids like anthocyanins, which have been linked to numerous health benefits, including improved cognitive function and heart health.

- Raspberries: Raspberries are small, delicate berries with a sweet-tart flavor and a rich source of dietary fiber, vitamins C and K, and antioxidants such as ellagic acid and quercetin. They come in various colors, including red, black, purple, and gold.

- Blackberries: Blackberries are similar in appearance to raspberries but have a darker color and a sweeter, juicier flavor. They are high in fiber, vitamin C, vitamin K, and manganese, as well as antioxidants like anthocyanins and ellagic acid.

- Cranberries: These tart, red berries are commonly consumed in dried or juice form and are known for their potential benefits for urinary tract health. Cranberries are rich in vitamin C, fiber, and antioxidants called proanthocyanidins, which may help prevent urinary tract infections (UTIs) by preventing bacteria from adhering to the urinary tract lining.

- Goji Berries: Also known as wolfberries, goji berries are small, red-orange berries native to Asia. They are prized for their high antioxidant content and are believed to have various health benefits, including boosting immune function, promoting eye health, and supporting skin health.

- Acai Berries: Acai berries are small, dark purple berries native to the Amazon rainforest and are often consumed in juice or powder form. They are rich in antioxidants, particularly anthocyanins and flavonoids, and are touted for their potential anti-inflammatory and heart-healthy effects.

2. Nutritional Composition:

- Berries are nutrient-dense foods, meaning they provide a high concentration of vitamins, minerals, antioxidants, and dietary fiber relative to their calorie content.

- Berries are particularly rich in vitamin C, an essential nutrient that plays a critical role in immune function, collagen synthesis, and antioxidant defense. They also contain significant amounts of vitamin K, manganese, and various B vitamins.

- Berries are among the richest sources of dietary antioxidants, including flavonoids, anthocyanins, polyphenols, and ellagic acid.

These antioxidants help protect cells and tissues from oxidative damage caused by free radicals and may reduce the risk of chronic diseases such as heart disease, cancer, and neurodegenerative disorders.

- The dietary fiber found in berries, particularly soluble fiber, helps promote digestive health, regulate blood sugar levels, and support weight management by increasing feelings of fullness and satiety.

3. Health Benefits:

- Antioxidant Protection: The high antioxidant content of berries helps neutralize free radicals and reduce oxidative stress in the body, which can help protect against chronic diseases and age-related decline.

- Heart Health: Berries have been associated with various cardiovascular benefits, including reducing LDL (bad) cholesterol levels, improving blood vessel function, and lowering blood pressure. The flavonoids and anthocyanins in berries may help prevent atherosclerosis and reduce the risk of heart disease and stroke.

- Cognitive Function: Some studies suggest that regular consumption of berries, particularly blueberries, may help improve cognitive function, memory, and executive function in older adults. The antioxidants and phytochemicals in berries may protect brain cells from oxidative damage and inflammation, potentially reducing the risk of age-related cognitive decline and neurodegenerative diseases like Alzheimer's disease.

- Blood Sugar Control: The fiber and antioxidants in berries can help regulate blood sugar levels and improve insulin sensitivity, making them beneficial for individuals with diabetes or at risk of developing type 2 diabetes. Berries have a low glycemic index and are less likely to cause spikes in blood sugar compared to high-glycemic foods.

- Anti-Inflammatory Effects: Some studies suggest that the bioactive compounds in berries, including anthocyanins, flavonoids, and ellagic acid, possess anti-inflammatory properties and may help reduce inflammation in the body. Chronic inflammation is linked to various health conditions, including heart disease, diabetes, and arthritis.

4. Culinary Uses:

- Berries are incredibly versatile and can be enjoyed in a variety of ways, both fresh and prepared. They can be eaten plain as a healthy snack or incorporated into a wide range of recipes, including:

- Smoothies and smoothie bowls
- Breakfast dishes such as oatmeal, yogurt parfaits, and pancakes
- Salads, both sweet and savory
- Desserts such as pies, cobblers, crisps, and fruit salads
- Baked goods like muffins, cakes, and tarts

- Sauces, jams, and preserves

5. Selection and Storage:

- When selecting fresh berries, look for plump, brightly colored fruits that are firm and free from mold or bruises. Avoid berries that are soft, mushy, or overly ripe.

- Store fresh berries in the refrigerator, preferably in a perforated container or paper towel-lined tray to allow air circulation and prevent moisture buildup. Berries are best consumed within a few days of purchase but can be frozen for longer-term storage.

- Frozen berries are a convenient option for enjoying berries out of season or for use in smoothies, baked goods, and other recipes. They can be kept in the freezer for several months and thawed as needed.

6. Cautions and Considerations:

- While berries are generally safe for most people to consume, some individuals may be allergic to certain types of berries or may experience digestive discomfort when consuming large quantities of fiber-rich berries.

- It's essential to wash fresh berries thoroughly before consumption to remove any dirt, pesticides, or bacteria that may be present on the skin.

- When consuming cranberry products like juice or supplements for urinary tract health, be sure to choose unsweetened options to avoid excess sugar intake.

In summary, berries are not only delicious but also nutrient-packed powerhouses that offer a wide range of health benefits. Whether enjoyed fresh, frozen, or incorporated into recipes, berries are a versatile and flavorful addition to any diet. By including a variety of berries in your meals and snacks, you can boost your intake of essential nutrients, support your overall health and well-being, and indulge in the natural sweetness and vibrant colors of these delightful fruits.

Cruciferous Vegetables

Cruciferous vegetables belong to the Brassicaceae family and are characterized by their cross-shaped flowers, from which they derive their name. These nutrient-rich vegetables are known for their unique flavors, textures, and health-promoting properties. Common cruciferous vegetables include broccoli, cauliflower, cabbage, Brussels sprouts, kale, collard greens, bok choy, and arugula. Let's explore the diverse aspects of cruciferous vegetables:

1. Nutritional Composition:
   - Cruciferous vegetables are packed with essential nutrients, including vitamins, minerals, fiber, and phytochemicals.

- They are rich in vitamin C, an antioxidant that supports immune function, collagen synthesis, and wound healing.

- Cruciferous vegetables are excellent sources of vitamin K, which is essential for blood clotting and bone health.

- They also contain significant amounts of folate (vitamin B9), potassium, manganese, and various B vitamins.

- Cruciferous vegetables are low in calories and carbohydrates, making them an excellent choice for those looking to manage their weight or blood sugar levels.

2. Health Benefits:

- Cancer Prevention: Cruciferous vegetables are renowned for their potential cancer-fighting properties. They contain sulfur-containing compounds called glucosinolates, which can be converted into bioactive compounds like isothiocyanates and indole-3-carbinol. These compounds have been shown to inhibit cancer cell growth, promote apoptosis (cell death), and reduce inflammation. Studies suggest that regular consumption of cruciferous vegetables may lower the risk of various cancers, including lung, breast, prostate, colorectal, and stomach cancer.

- Heart Health: The fiber, antioxidants, and phytochemicals found in cruciferous vegetables may help reduce the risk of heart disease by lowering LDL (bad) cholesterol levels, improving blood vessel function, and reducing inflammation. Cruciferous vegetables are also rich in potassium, which supports healthy blood pressure levels and cardiovascular function.

- Digestive Health: The fiber content of cruciferous vegetables promotes digestive health by supporting regular bowel movements, preventing constipation, and feeding beneficial gut bacteria. Fiber also helps regulate blood sugar levels and may reduce the risk of digestive disorders like diverticulosis and hemorrhoids.

- Bone Health: Cruciferous vegetables are excellent sources of vitamin K, which is essential for bone health and calcium metabolism. Adequate vitamin K intake may help prevent osteoporosis and reduce the risk of fractures by supporting bone mineralization and density.

- Detoxification: Certain compounds found in cruciferous vegetables, such as sulforaphane, have been shown to support detoxification pathways in the body, particularly in the liver. These compounds may help neutralize harmful toxins, pollutants, and carcinogens, aiding in the body's natural detoxification process.

- Anti-Inflammatory Effects: The phytochemicals and antioxidants in cruciferous vegetables have anti-inflammatory properties that may help reduce inflammation in the body. Chronic inflammation is linked to various health conditions, including heart disease, diabetes, arthritis, and cancer.

3. Culinary Uses:

- Cruciferous vegetables can be enjoyed in a variety of ways, both raw and cooked. They add flavor, texture, and nutritional value to a wide range of dishes, including salads, stir-fries, soups, stews, casseroles, and side dishes.

- When cooking cruciferous vegetables, it's important not to overcook them, as prolonged cooking can lead to nutrient loss and a mushy texture. Steaming, sautéing, roasting, and blanching are popular cooking methods that help retain the vegetables' natural flavors, colors, and nutrients.

- Raw cruciferous vegetables can be enjoyed in salads, slaws, wraps, and sandwiches, providing a crunchy texture and refreshing taste.

4. Varieties and Preparation:

- Broccoli: Known for its green, tree-like florets, broccoli is one of the most versatile and widely consumed cruciferous vegetables. It can be steamed, roasted, stir-fried, or enjoyed raw in salads or crudité platters.

- Cauliflower: Cauliflower is prized for its mild flavor and versatile culinary applications. It can be mashed, riced, roasted, grilled, or used as a low-carb alternative to grains and starches in dishes like cauliflower rice, cauliflower pizza crust, and cauliflower mashed potatoes.

- Cabbage: Cabbage comes in various colors, including green, red, and Napa (Chinese) cabbage. It can be used in salads, coleslaws, stir-fries, soups, stews, and fermented foods like sauerkraut and kimchi.

- **Brussels Sprouts**: Brussels sprouts are small, cabbage-like vegetables that grow on stalks. They can be roasted, sautéed, grilled, or shaved raw in salads.

- Kale: Kale is a nutrient-dense leafy green vegetable with a slightly bitter taste. It can be used in salads, smoothies, soups, stews, and sautés, or baked into crispy kale chips.

- Collard Greens: Collard greens are large, leafy greens commonly used in Southern cuisine. They can be braised, boiled, sautéed, or used as a wrap for sandwiches or burritos.

- Bok Choy: Bok choy, also known as Chinese cabbage, has tender, white stalks and dark green leaves. It can be stir-fried, steamed, sautéed, or added to soups and stir-fries for a mild, slightly sweet flavor.

5. Selection and Storage:

- When selecting cruciferous vegetables, choose those that are firm, dense, and free from blemishes or signs of decay. The leaves should be vibrant and crisp, with no wilting or yellowing.

- Store cruciferous vegetables in the refrigerator in a perforated plastic bag or vegetable crisper drawer to maintain freshness and prevent moisture buildup. Most cruciferous vegetables will keep for several days to a week when stored properly.

- Wash cruciferous vegetables thoroughly before use, particularly if they will be consumed raw, to remove any dirt, bacteria, or pesticide residues.

In summary, cruciferous vegetables are nutritional powerhouses that offer a wide range of health benefits and culinary possibilities. By incorporating a variety of cruciferous vegetables into your meals and snacks, you can enjoy their delicious flavors, vibrant colors, and numerous health-promoting properties. Whether enjoyed raw or cooked, cruciferous vegetables are a tasty and nutritious addition to any diet, supporting overall health and well-being.

Whole Grains

Whole grains are a vital component of a healthy diet, offering a plethora of nutrients, fiber, and health benefits. Unlike refined grains, which have been stripped of their bran and germ during processing, whole grains contain all parts of the grain kernel, including the bran, germ, and endosperm. This means they retain the natural nutrients, fiber, and antioxidants found in the grain, making them a nutritious and wholesome choice. Let's delve into the diverse aspects of whole grains:

1. Varieties of Whole Grains:

- Wheat: Whole wheat is perhaps the most well-known whole grain, available in various forms such as whole wheat flour, bulgur, farro, and wheat berries.

- Oats: Oats are a versatile whole grain commonly consumed as oatmeal, rolled oats, steel-cut oats, or oat groats. They are rich in soluble fiber, particularly beta-glucan, which helps lower cholesterol levels and promote digestive health.

- Brown Rice: Brown rice is a whole grain rice variety that retains its bran and germ layers, providing more fiber, vitamins, and minerals compared to white rice. It comes in long, medium, and short grain varieties and can be used in a wide range of dishes.

- Quinoa: Quinoa is a pseudo-grain technically classified as a seed, but it is often referred to as a whole grain due to its similar culinary uses and nutritional profile. It is prized for its high protein content, complete amino acid profile, and gluten-free status.

- Barley: Barley is a hearty whole grain with a nutty flavor and chewy texture. It can be used in soups, stews, salads, and pilafs, providing fiber, vitamins, and minerals such as manganese and selenium.

- Buckwheat: Despite its name, buckwheat is not a type of wheat and is naturally gluten-free. It is commonly consumed as buckwheat groats, flour, or noodles and is rich in protein, fiber, and antioxidants like rutin.

- Millet: Millet is a small, gluten-free grain with a mildly sweet flavor and fluffy texture when cooked. It is a staple food in many parts of the world and can be used in porridges, pilafs, and baked goods.

- Amaranth: Amaranth is a tiny seed that is often classified as a pseudo-grain due to its culinary uses and nutritional profile. It is gluten-free and rich in protein, fiber, and micronutrients like iron and magnesium.

2. Nutritional Composition:

- Whole grains are nutrient-dense foods, providing essential nutrients such as complex carbohydrates, dietary fiber, protein, vitamins, minerals, and antioxidants.

- They are rich in complex carbohydrates, which serve as the primary source of energy for the body and help maintain stable blood sugar levels.

- Whole grains are excellent sources of dietary fiber, including both soluble and insoluble fiber, which promote digestive health, regulate bowel movements, and support weight management by increasing feelings of fullness and satiety.

- They are also rich in B vitamins, including thiamine (B1), riboflavin (B2), niacin (B3), pantothenic acid (B5), pyridoxine (B6), and folate (B9), which play vital roles in energy metabolism, nerve function, red blood cell production, and DNA synthesis.

- Whole grains contain essential minerals such as iron, magnesium, phosphorus, zinc, and selenium, which are important for bone health, muscle function, immune function, and overall well-being.

- Additionally, whole grains are rich in antioxidants, including phenolic compounds, lignans, and tocopherols, which help protect cells and tissues from oxidative damage caused by free radicals.

3. Health Benefits:

- Heart Health: Whole grains have been associated with numerous cardiovascular benefits, including reducing the risk of heart disease, stroke, and hypertension. The fiber, antioxidants, and phytochemicals found in whole grains help lower LDL (bad) cholesterol levels, improve blood vessel function, and reduce inflammation.

- Digestive Health: The dietary fiber in whole grains promotes digestive health by preventing constipation, regulating bowel movements, and feeding beneficial gut bacteria. Whole grains may help reduce the risk of digestive disorders such as diverticulosis, hemorrhoids, and colorectal cancer.

- Weight Management: Whole grains can support weight management by promoting satiety, reducing calorie intake, and stabilizing blood sugar levels. The fiber and protein in whole grains help keep you feeling full and satisfied, preventing overeating and snacking between meals.

- Blood Sugar Control: The fiber, protein, and complex carbohydrates in whole grains help slow down the absorption of sugar into the bloodstream, preventing spikes and crashes in blood sugar levels. Whole grains have a lower glycemic index compared to refined grains, making them a better choice for individuals with diabetes or insulin resistance.

- Reduced Risk of Chronic Diseases: Regular consumption of whole grains has been linked to a reduced risk of chronic diseases such as type 2 diabetes, certain cancers (e.g., colorectal cancer), and neurodegenerative disorders like Alzheimer's disease. The antioxidants and phytochemicals in whole grains help protect cells and tissues from damage and inflammation associated with these conditions.

- Longevity: Some studies suggest that a diet rich in whole grains may contribute to longevity and overall well-being by reducing the risk of premature death from cardiovascular disease, cancer, and other chronic diseases.

4. Culinary Uses:

- Whole grains can be incorporated into a wide range of dishes, including breakfast foods, salads, soups, stews, pilafs, casseroles, and baked goods.

- They can be cooked and served as a side dish, mixed with vegetables and proteins for a main course, or used as a base for grain bowls and salads.

- Whole grain flours can be used in baking to make bread, muffins, pancakes, waffles, cookies, and other baked goods. They can also be used as thickeners for sauces and gravies.

5. Selection and Storage:

- When selecting whole grains, look for intact grains that are clean, dry, and free from signs of moisture, mold, or insect damage. Avoid grains that appear discolored, dusty, or have a rancid smell.

- Store whole grains in a cool, dry place in airtight containers to protect them from moisture, pests, and oxidation. Some whole grains, such as brown rice and oats, may benefit from refrigeration or freezing to prolong shelf life and maintain freshness.

In summary, whole grains are an essential component of a balanced diet, providing a wide range of nutrients, fiber, and health benefits. By incorporating a variety of whole grains into your meals and snacks, you can enjoy their delicious flavors, textures, and nutritional benefits while supporting your overall health and well-being. Whether enjoyed as a hearty side dish, wholesome breakfast, or satisfying snack, whole grains are a versatile and nutritious addition to any diet.

Nuts and Seeds

Nuts and seeds are nutrient-dense foods that offer a wealth of health benefits, including essential nutrients, healthy fats, protein, fiber, and antioxidants. They come in a variety of shapes, sizes, flavors, and textures, making them versatile additions to a balanced diet. From almonds and walnuts to chia seeds and flaxseeds, nuts and seeds are prized for their nutritional value and culinary versatility. Let's explore the diverse aspects of nuts and seeds:

1. Varieties of Nuts:

- Almonds: Almonds are one of the most popular and widely consumed nuts, prized for their delicate flavor, crunchy texture, and numerous health benefits. They are rich in vitamin E, magnesium, calcium, and healthy fats, particularly monounsaturated fats.

- Walnuts: Walnuts are known for their distinctively shaped shells and brain-like appearance. They are a rich source of omega-3 fatty acids, antioxidants, and polyphenols, which have been linked to various health benefits, including heart health and brain function.

- Cashews: Cashews are kidney-shaped nuts with a buttery texture and mild, sweet flavor. They are rich in minerals such as copper, magnesium, and zinc, as well as healthy fats and protein.

- Pistachios: Pistachios are small, green nuts with a slightly sweet and savory flavor. They are rich in protein, fiber, potassium, and antioxidants like lutein and zeaxanthin, which are beneficial for eye health.

- Hazelnuts: Hazelnuts, also known as filberts, are small, round nuts with a sweet, nutty flavor. They are rich in vitamin E, folate, and healthy fats, particularly monounsaturated fats.

- Brazil Nuts: Brazil nuts are large, crescent-shaped nuts native to South America. They are a good source of selenium, a trace mineral with antioxidant properties that support immune function and thyroid health.

- Pecans: Pecans are native to North America and have a rich, buttery flavor. They are high in healthy fats, fiber, and antioxidants like vitamin E and ellagic acid, which may help reduce inflammation and oxidative stress.

- Macadamia Nuts: Macadamia nuts are creamy, buttery nuts native to Australia. They are high in monounsaturated fats, particularly oleic acid, which may help lower LDL (bad) cholesterol levels and reduce the risk of heart disease.

2. Varieties of Seeds:

- Chia Seeds: Chia seeds are tiny black or white seeds native to Mexico and Central America. They are rich in fiber, protein, omega-3 fatty acids, and antioxidants, making them a nutritious addition to smoothies, oatmeal, and baked goods.

- Flaxseeds: Flaxseeds, also known as linseeds, are small, brown seeds with a nutty flavor. They are a rich source of alpha-linolenic acid (ALA), a type of omega-3 fatty acid, as well as lignans, fiber, and protein.

- Sunflower Seeds: Sunflower seeds are the edible seeds of the sunflower plant, prized for their mild, nutty flavor and crunchy texture. They are rich in vitamin E, selenium, magnesium, and healthy fats, particularly linoleic acid.

- Pumpkin Seeds: Pumpkin seeds, also known as pepitas, are flat, green seeds found inside pumpkin or squash fruits. They are a good source of protein, iron, zinc, magnesium, and antioxidants like vitamin E and carotenoids.

- Sesame Seeds: Sesame seeds are small, flat seeds with a rich, nutty flavor commonly used in cooking and baking. They are a good source of calcium, magnesium, iron, zinc, and healthy fats.

- Hemp Seeds: Hemp seeds are small, creamy white seeds derived from the hemp plant. They are rich in protein, omega-3 and omega-6 fatty acids, fiber, and antioxidants, making them a nutritious addition to salads, smoothies, and baked goods.

3. Nutritional Composition:

- Nuts and seeds are nutrient powerhouses, providing a wide range of essential nutrients, including vitamins, minerals, protein, healthy fats, fiber, and antioxidants.

- They are rich in monounsaturated and polyunsaturated fats, including omega-3 and omega-6 fatty acids, which are essential for brain health, heart health, and overall well-being.

- Nuts and seeds are excellent sources of plant-based protein, making them ideal for vegetarians, vegans, and individuals looking to reduce their intake of animal products.

- They are also rich in fiber, both soluble and insoluble, which promotes digestive health, regulates bowel movements, and helps keep you feeling full and satisfied.

- Nuts and seeds are rich in vitamins and minerals, including vitamin E, magnesium, calcium, phosphorus, potassium, zinc, and iron, which play vital roles in various physiological processes, such as immune function, bone health, and energy metabolism.

- Additionally, nuts and seeds are packed with antioxidants, including vitamin E, selenium, flavonoids, and polyphenols, which help protect cells and tissues from oxidative damage caused by free radicals.

4. Health Benefits:

- Heart Health: Nuts and seeds have been associated with numerous cardiovascular benefits, including reducing LDL (bad) cholesterol levels, improving blood vessel function, and lowering the risk of heart disease and stroke. The monounsaturated and polyunsaturated fats in nuts and seeds help lower blood pressure, reduce inflammation, and improve lipid profiles.

- Weight Management: Despite their high calorie and fat content, nuts and seeds can support weight management when consumed in moderation. The protein, fiber, and healthy fats in nuts and seeds help increase feelings of fullness and satiety, reducing overall calorie intake and preventing overeating.

- Blood Sugar Control: The protein, fiber, and healthy fats in nuts and seeds help slow down the absorption of sugar into the bloodstream, preventing spikes and crashes in blood sugar levels. Including nuts and seeds in meals and snacks can help stabilize blood sugar levels and reduce the risk of insulin resistance and type 2 diabetes.

- Brain Health: The omega-3 fatty acids found in certain nuts and seeds, such as walnuts, flaxseeds, and chia seeds, are essential for brain health and cognitive function. They help support neuronal structure and function, improve memory and learning, and may reduce the risk of age-related cognitive decline and neurodegenerative diseases like Alzheimer's disease.

- Digestive Health: The fiber content of nuts and seeds promotes digestive health by supporting regular bowel movements, preventing constipation, and feeding beneficial gut bacteria. Including nuts and seeds in your diet can help maintain a healthy gut microbiome and reduce the risk of digestive disorders like diverticulosis and hemorrhoids.

- Bone Health: Nuts and seeds are rich in minerals such as calcium, magnesium, phosphorus, and zinc, which are important for bone health and density. Including nuts and seeds in your diet can help support bone growth, maintenance, and repair, reducing the risk of osteoporosis and fractures.

5. Culinary Uses:

- Nuts and seeds can be enjoyed in a variety of ways, both raw and roasted, and can be incorporated into a wide range of dishes, including salads, stir-fries, soups, stews, baked goods, granolas, trail mixes, and nut butters.

- They can be sprinkled over oatmeal, yogurt, or smoothie bowls for added texture and flavor, or used as toppings for salads, vegetables, and grain bowls.

- Nuts and seeds can be ground into flours and used as gluten-free alternatives in baking, or blended into creamy nut and seed butters for spreads, dips, and sauces.

- They can also be used as crunchy coatings for meats, fish, and tofu, or ground into pestos, sauces, and dressings for added flavor and nutrition.

6. Selection and Storage:

- When selecting nuts and seeds, look for those that are fresh, dry, and free from signs of mold, rancidity, or insect damage. Avoid nuts and seeds that appear discolored, shriveled, or have an off smell.

- Store nuts and seeds in a cool, dry place away from heat, light, and moisture to prevent them from becoming stale or rancid. Airtight containers or resealable bags are ideal for storing nuts and seeds.

- Some nuts and seeds, particularly those high in unsaturated fats like omega-3 fatty acids, are more prone to rancidity and should be stored in the refrigerator or freezer to prolong shelf life and maintain freshness.

In summary, nuts and seeds are nutrient-rich foods that offer a wide range of health benefits and culinary possibilities. By including a variety of nuts and seeds in your diet, you can enjoy their delicious flavors, textures, and nutritional benefits while supporting your overall health and well-being. Whether enjoyed as a convenient snack, wholesome ingredient, or flavorful topping, nuts and seeds are versatile additions to any diet, providing essential nutrients and promoting optimal health and vitality.

Chapter 5:

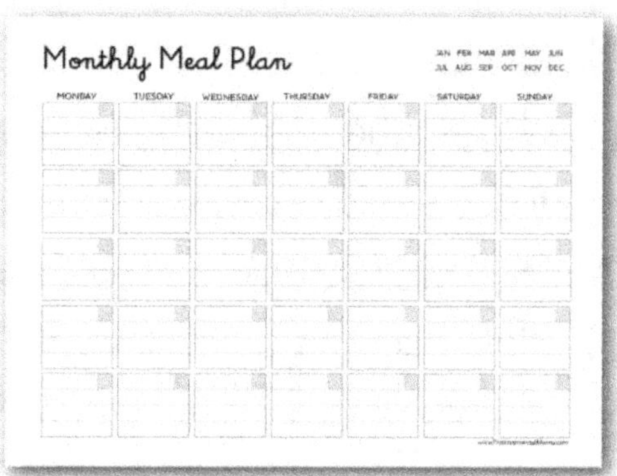

Meal Planning with Fat-Burning Foods

Meal planning with fat-burning foods involves strategic selection and preparation of ingredients that promote metabolism, satiety, and weight loss. By incorporating nutrient-dense foods that are rich in protein, fiber, healthy fats, vitamins, and minerals, you can create balanced meals that support fat burning and overall health. Here's a comprehensive guide to meal planning with fat-burning foods:

1. Understanding Fat-Burning Foods:

- Fat-burning foods are those that stimulate metabolism, increase energy expenditure, and promote fat loss when consumed as part of a balanced diet.

- These foods often have specific characteristics, such as being low in calories, high in nutrients, and containing compounds that enhance metabolic function.

- Examples of fat-burning foods include lean proteins like chicken breast, turkey, fish, tofu, and legumes; non-starchy vegetables such as leafy greens, broccoli, cauliflower, and bell peppers; whole grains like quinoa, brown rice, oats, and barley; healthy fats like avocado, nuts, seeds, and olive oil; and metabolism-boosting spices and herbs like cayenne pepper, ginger, cinnamon, and turmeric.

2. Setting Nutritional Goals:

- Before you start meal planning, it's essential to set specific nutritional goals based on your individual needs, preferences, and health objectives.

- Determine your daily calorie requirements based on factors such as age, gender, weight, height, activity level, and weight loss goals.

- Aim to create balanced meals that include a mix of macronutrients (protein, carbohydrates, and fats) and micronutrients (vitamins and minerals) to support overall health and well-being.

- Consider consulting with a registered dietitian or nutritionist to personalize your meal plan and ensure it aligns with your dietary preferences and nutritional needs.

3. Creating a Meal Plan:

- Start by planning your meals for the week ahead, taking into account your schedule, budget, and available ingredients.

- Choose a variety of fat-burning foods from different food groups to ensure you're getting a wide range of nutrients and flavors throughout the week.

- Incorporate lean proteins into each meal to support muscle maintenance, satiety, and metabolism. Opt for grilled chicken, baked fish, tofu stir-fry, lentil soup, or bean salads.

- Include plenty of non-starchy vegetables and leafy greens in your meals to add volume, fiber, and essential nutrients without excess calories. Experiment with colorful vegetables like spinach, kale, bell peppers, tomatoes, carrots, and cucumbers.

- Incorporate whole grains and complex carbohydrates to provide sustained energy and promote satiety. Choose options like quinoa, brown rice, whole wheat pasta, barley, or sweet potatoes.

- Don't forget to include healthy fats in your meals to enhance flavor, satiety, and nutrient absorption. Add sliced avocado to salads, sprinkle nuts and seeds on oatmeal or yogurt, or drizzle olive oil over roasted vegetables.

- Experiment with different cooking methods and flavor combinations to keep your meals interesting and satisfying. Try grilling, baking, sautéing, steaming, or roasting your proteins and vegetables with herbs, spices, and citrus zest for added flavor.

4. Batch Cooking and Meal Prep:

- Save time and streamline your meal planning process by batch cooking and meal prepping certain components of your meals in advance.

- Cook large batches of grains, proteins, and vegetables at the beginning of the week and portion them out into individual containers for easy grab-and-go meals.

- Prep ingredients like chopped vegetables, washed greens, cooked grains, and marinated proteins to assemble quick and nutritious meals throughout the week.

- Invest in quality food storage containers, reusable bags, and meal prep containers to keep your prepped ingredients fresh and organized in the refrigerator or freezer.

5. Balanced and Satisfying Meals:

- Aim to create balanced meals that include a mix of protein, carbohydrates, and fats, along with plenty of fiber-rich vegetables and leafy greens.

- Start your day with a protein-rich breakfast to kickstart your metabolism and keep you feeling full and energized throughout the morning. Try options like scrambled eggs with spinach and avocado, Greek yogurt with berries and almonds, or a smoothie made with protein powder, kale, and frozen fruit.

- For lunch and dinner, focus on filling half your plate with non-starchy vegetables, a quarter with lean protein, and a quarter with whole grains or starchy vegetables. Experiment with different flavor combinations and cuisines to keep your meals interesting and satisfying.

- Incorporate snacks into your meal plan to help curb hunger and prevent overeating at mealtimes. Choose nutrient-dense snacks like raw vegetables with hummus, Greek yogurt with fruit, or a small handful of nuts and seeds.

6. Portion Control and Mindful Eating:

- Practice portion control and mindful eating to avoid overeating and promote better digestion and satiety.

- Pay attention to hunger and fullness cues, eating slowly and savoring each bite. Stop eating when you feel comfortably satisfied rather than overly full.

- Use smaller plates, bowls, and utensils to help control portion sizes and prevent overeating. Aim to fill your plate with mostly vegetables and lean protein, with smaller portions of grains or starches and fats.

- Be mindful of portion sizes when eating out or dining at restaurants, as portion sizes tend to be larger than what you might serve yourself at home. Consider splitting meals with a dining companion or asking for a half portion if available.

7. Hydration and Beverage Choices:

- Stay hydrated throughout the day by drinking plenty of water, herbal teas, and other calorie-free beverages. Adequate hydration is essential for optimal metabolism, digestion, and fat burning.

- Limit your intake of sugary drinks, sodas, fruit juices, and alcoholic beverages, which can contribute to excess calorie consumption and hinder fat loss efforts.

- Consider incorporating metabolism-boosting beverages like green tea or matcha into your routine, as they contain catechins and caffeine, which may enhance fat oxidation and energy expenditure.

8. Tracking and Adjusting:

- Keep track of your meals, snacks, and hydration throughout the week to monitor your progress and identify areas for improvement.

- Use a food journal, meal planning app, or nutrition tracking tool to record what you eat, how much you eat, and how you feel after eating.

- Pay attention to how your body responds to different foods and meals, making adjustments as needed to better support your energy levels, hunger cues, and weight loss goals.

- Be patient and consistent with your meal planning efforts, recognizing that progress takes time and effort. Celebrate small victories along the way and stay focused on your long-term health and well-being.

In summary, meal planning with fat-burning foods involves thoughtful selection, preparation, and portioning of ingredients that support metabolism, satiety, and weight loss. By incorporating nutrient-dense foods like lean proteins, fiber-rich vegetables, whole grains, and healthy fats into your meals and snacks, you can create balanced and satisfying meals that promote fat burning and overall health. Experiment with different recipes, flavors, and cooking methods to keep your meals interesting and enjoyable while staying focused on your nutritional goals and objectives. With careful planning and mindful eating, you can fuel your body with the nutrients it needs to thrive and achieve your desired health outcomes.

Breakfast Options

Breakfast is often hailed as the most important meal of the day, and for good reason. It provides the fuel your body needs to kickstart your metabolism, replenish energy stores after a night of fasting, and set the tone for your day ahead. Opting for nutrient-dense breakfast options can help you feel satisfied, energized, and focused until your next meal. Here's a comprehensive guide to breakfast options that are both delicious and nutritious:

1. Importance of Breakfast:

- Breakfast literally means "breaking the fast," as it is the first meal consumed after a period of overnight fasting.

- Eating breakfast jumpstarts your metabolism, helping your body burn calories more efficiently throughout the day.

- Breakfast provides essential nutrients such as carbohydrates, protein, healthy fats, fiber, vitamins, and minerals, which are vital for optimal health and well-being.

- Consuming breakfast has been linked to numerous health benefits, including improved cognitive function, better concentration and memory, enhanced mood, and reduced risk of obesity and chronic diseases.

2. Components of a Balanced Breakfast:

- Protein: Incorporating protein into your breakfast helps promote satiety, stabilize blood sugar levels, and support muscle repair and growth. Good sources of protein include eggs, Greek yogurt, cottage cheese, tofu, tempeh, smoked salmon, turkey bacon, and protein powder.

- Carbohydrates: Choose complex carbohydrates that provide sustained energy and fiber to keep you feeling full and satisfied. Whole grains like oats, quinoa, barley, whole wheat bread, and brown rice are excellent options. You can also include fruits such as berries, bananas, apples, and citrus fruits for natural sweetness and additional nutrients.

- Healthy Fats: Adding healthy fats to your breakfast helps enhance flavor, promote satiety, and support nutrient absorption. Avocado, nuts, seeds, nut butter, coconut oil, and olive oil are all great choices for incorporating healthy fats into your morning meal.

- Fiber: Fiber-rich foods like fruits, vegetables, whole grains, nuts, and seeds are essential for digestive health, bowel regularity, and weight management. Aim to include fiber in your breakfast to promote feelings of fullness and support overall gut health.

- Vitamins and Minerals: Choose a variety of colorful fruits and vegetables to ensure you're getting a wide range of vitamins, minerals, and antioxidants in your breakfast. Leafy greens, bell peppers, tomatoes, berries, and citrus fruits are excellent sources of essential nutrients.

3. Breakfast Options:

- Classic Breakfast Staples:

- Scrambled or poached eggs with whole grain toast and sliced avocado.

- Greek yogurt parfait with granola, berries, and a drizzle of honey or maple syrup.

- Oatmeal topped with sliced banana, almond butter, and a sprinkle of cinnamon.

- Whole grain pancakes or waffles topped with Greek yogurt and fresh fruit.

- Breakfast burrito or wrap filled with scrambled eggs, black beans, salsa, and avocado.

- Smoothie Bowls:

- Green smoothie bowl made with spinach, kale, banana, pineapple, and coconut water, topped with sliced almonds, shredded coconut, and chia seeds.

- Berry smoothie bowl made with mixed berries, Greek yogurt, almond milk, and protein powder, topped with granola, sliced strawberries, and hemp seeds.

- Tropical smoothie bowl made with mango, pineapple, coconut milk, and spinach, topped with toasted coconut flakes, sliced kiwi, and pumpkin seeds.

- Egg-Based Dishes:

- Veggie-packed omelet or frittata filled with spinach, mushrooms, bell peppers, onions, and feta cheese.

- Breakfast sandwich with whole grain English muffin, scrambled eggs, turkey sausage or bacon, and sliced tomato.

- Quiche or crustless mini quiches made with eggs, broccoli, sun-dried tomatoes, and goat cheese.

- Grab-and-Go Options:

- Overnight oats prepared with rolled oats, chia seeds, almond milk, and mixed berries, topped with sliced almonds and a drizzle of honey.

- Homemade breakfast bars or energy balls made with oats, nuts, seeds, dried fruit, and nut butter.

- Whole grain muffins or scones packed with nuts, seeds, and fruit for a portable breakfast option.

- Protein-packed smoothies made with spinach, banana, protein powder, almond milk, and nut butter for a quick and convenient breakfast on busy mornings.

4. Customization and Variation:

- Get creative with your breakfast options by experimenting with different flavor combinations, ingredients, and cooking techniques.

- Mix and match your favorite ingredients to create custom breakfast bowls, sandwiches, wraps, or salads that suit your taste preferences and dietary needs.

- Don't be afraid to think outside the box and try new foods or recipes to keep your breakfast routine exciting and enjoyable.

- Consider batch cooking or meal prepping certain components of your breakfasts, such as overnight oats, breakfast muffins, or smoothie packs, to save time during the week.

5. Timing and Frequency:

- Aim to eat breakfast within an hour or two of waking up to replenish energy stores and jumpstart your metabolism.

- Listen to your body's hunger cues and eat breakfast when you feel hungry, rather than forcing yourself to eat if you're not hungry first thing in the morning.

- If you're not typically hungry in the morning, start with a small, light breakfast and gradually increase the size and complexity of your morning meal as your appetite increases.

6. Hydration and Beverage Choices:

- Pair your breakfast with a glass of water or herbal tea to stay hydrated and promote optimal digestion.

- Limit your intake of sugary beverages like fruit juice, soda, and flavored coffee drinks, which can contribute to excess calorie consumption and blood sugar spikes.

- Opt for unsweetened beverages like black coffee, green tea, or sparkling water with lemon to accompany your breakfast and support your overall health and hydration needs.

In summary, breakfast is an essential meal that sets the tone for your day and provides the fuel your body needs to function optimally. By choosing nutrient-dense breakfast options that include a mix of protein, carbohydrates, healthy fats, fiber, vitamins, and minerals, you can support your metabolism, energy levels, and overall well-being. Experiment with different breakfast recipes, flavors, and ingredients to find what works best for you, and don't forget to listen to your body's hunger cues and eat breakfast when you feel hungry and ready to start your day on the right foot.

Lunch Ideas

Lunch is an important meal that provides the opportunity to refuel your body and mind halfway through the day. Choosing nutrient-dense lunch options can help sustain energy levels, boost productivity, and support overall health and well-being. Whether you're meal prepping at home, grabbing lunch on the go, or enjoying a midday meal at a restaurant, there are plenty of delicious and nutritious options to consider. Here's a comprehensive guide to lunch ideas that are both satisfying and nourishing:

1. Components of a Balanced Lunch:

- Protein: Including a source of protein in your lunch helps promote satiety, support muscle repair and growth, and stabilize blood sugar levels. Choose lean proteins such as grilled chicken breast, turkey, tofu, tempeh, beans, lentils, chickpeas, or fish like salmon or tuna.

- Vegetables: Load up on non-starchy vegetables and leafy greens to add volume, fiber, and essential nutrients to your lunch. Aim to fill at least half your plate with colorful vegetables such as spinach, kale, broccoli, bell peppers, carrots, cucumbers, tomatoes, and zucchini.

- Whole Grains: Incorporating complex carbohydrates from whole grains helps provide sustained energy and promotes feelings of fullness and satisfaction. Opt for options like brown rice, quinoa, barley, farro, whole wheat pasta, whole grain bread, or ancient grains like bulgur or freekeh.

- Healthy Fats: Including sources of healthy fats in your lunch adds flavor, richness, and satiety while supporting nutrient absorption and brain health. Add avocado slices, nuts, seeds, olives, or a drizzle of olive oil or tahini to your salads, sandwiches, or grain bowls.

- Flavor Enhancers: Boost the flavor and enjoyment of your lunch with herbs, spices, condiments, and sauces. Experiment with different combinations of herbs like basil, cilantro, parsley, and mint, as well as spices like garlic, ginger, cumin, paprika, and turmeric. Dress salads with vinaigrettes, pestos, or yogurt-based sauces, and use condiments like mustard, hummus, salsa, or tzatziki to add depth and complexity to your meals.

2. Lunch Ideas:

- Salads:

- Greek salad with mixed greens, cucumber, tomato, red onion, olives, feta cheese, and grilled chicken, drizzled with olive oil and balsamic vinegar.

- Cobb salad with mixed greens, hard-boiled eggs, avocado, cherry tomatoes, bacon bits, grilled chicken, and blue cheese, served with a creamy vinaigrette dressing.

- Quinoa salad with roasted vegetables, chickpeas, feta cheese, fresh herbs, and a lemon tahini dressing.

- Asian-inspired salad with mixed greens, shredded cabbage, carrots, bell peppers, edamame, grilled tofu or shrimp, and a sesame ginger dressing.

- Sandwiches and Wraps:

- Turkey avocado wrap with whole grain tortilla, sliced turkey breast, avocado, lettuce, tomato, and mustard.

- Veggie hummus sandwich on whole grain bread with hummus, sliced cucumber, bell pepper, shredded carrots, sprouts, and avocado.

- Caprese panini with whole grain bread, sliced tomato, fresh mozzarella, basil leaves, and balsamic glaze, pressed until crispy and melted.

- Tuna salad sandwich on whole grain bread with canned tuna, Greek yogurt, diced celery, red onion, and Dijon mustard.

- **Grain Bowls:**

- Mediterranean grain bowl with cooked quinoa, roasted vegetables (eggplant, zucchini, bell peppers), cherry tomatoes, olives, feta cheese, and grilled chicken or falafel, drizzled with tzatziki sauce.

- Teriyaki tofu bowl with brown rice, stir-fried vegetables (broccoli, bell peppers, snap peas), marinated tofu, sliced avocado, and a drizzle of teriyaki sauce.

- Burrito bowl with brown rice, black beans, grilled chicken or beef, sautéed peppers and onions, diced tomatoes, shredded lettuce, avocado slices, and salsa.

- Harvest grain bowl with cooked farro, roasted butternut squash, Brussels sprouts, cranberries, pecans, goat cheese, and a maple balsamic dressing.

- **Soups and Stews:**

- Chicken vegetable soup with shredded chicken, carrots, celery, onion, garlic, spinach, and quinoa in a savory broth.

- Lentil and vegetable stew with brown lentils, diced tomatoes, carrots, celery, onion, garlic, kale, and herbs, served with a slice of whole grain bread.

- Minestrone soup with cannellini beans, zucchini, tomatoes, carrots, celery, pasta, and fresh herbs in a flavorful broth.

- Thai coconut curry soup with tofu or shrimp, bell peppers, snap peas, carrots, mushrooms, and rice noodles in a creamy coconut curry broth.

- Leftovers:

- Utilize leftovers from dinner the night before to create quick and convenient lunches. Repurpose grilled chicken, roasted vegetables, cooked grains, or stir-fries into salads, wraps, bowls, or soups for a satisfying midday meal.

3. Customization and Variation:

- Mix and match ingredients and flavors to create custom lunch options that suit your taste preferences, dietary needs, and seasonal availability.

- Experiment with different protein sources, vegetables, grains, and flavor profiles to keep your lunches interesting and enjoyable.

- Get creative with leftovers, meal prep ingredients, and pantry staples to minimize food waste and maximize convenience.

4. Portion Control and Mindful Eating:

- Pay attention to portion sizes and serving sizes to avoid overeating and support weight management and digestion.

- Eat slowly, savoring each bite, and listen to your body's hunger and fullness cues to guide your eating patterns.

- Avoid distractions while eating, such as eating at your desk or in front of the TV, and focus on the sensory experience of enjoying your meal.

5. Hydration and Beverage Choices:

- Pair your lunch with a refreshing beverage like water, sparkling water, herbal tea, or unsweetened iced tea to stay hydrated and support digestion.

- Limit your intake of sugary drinks, sodas, and alcoholic beverages, which can add unnecessary calories and contribute to dehydration and fatigue.

In summary, lunch is an important opportunity to refuel your body and mind with nutrient-dense foods that support energy, productivity, and overall health and well-being. By choosing balanced lunch options that include a mix of protein, vegetables, whole grains, healthy fats, and flavor enhancers, you can create satisfying and nourishing meals that keep you fueled and satisfied throughout the day. Experiment with different recipes, ingredients, and flavor combinations to find what works best for you, and don't forget to prioritize portion control, mindful eating, and hydration for optimal health and wellness.

Dinner Recipes

Dinner is often considered the main meal of the day, providing an opportunity to unwind, connect with loved ones, and nourish your body with a satisfying and nutritious meal. Whether you're cooking for yourself, your family, or guests, dinner can be a time to get creative in the kitchen and explore a variety of flavors, ingredients, and cuisines. Here's a comprehensive guide to dinner recipes that are both delicious and nourishing:

1. Components of a Balanced Dinner:

   - Protein: Including a source of lean protein in your dinner helps support muscle repair and growth, promote satiety, and stabilize blood sugar levels. Choose options such as poultry (chicken, turkey), fish (salmon, trout, tilapia), seafood (shrimp, scallops), tofu, tempeh, beans, lentils, or legumes.

- Vegetables: Load up on colorful vegetables to add fiber, vitamins, minerals, and antioxidants to your dinner. Aim to fill at least half your plate with non-starchy vegetables such as leafy greens, cruciferous vegetables (broccoli, cauliflower, Brussels sprouts), bell peppers, carrots, zucchini, eggplant, and tomatoes.

- Whole Grains: Incorporating complex carbohydrates from whole grains helps provide sustained energy and promotes feelings of fullness and satisfaction. Choose options like brown rice, quinoa, barley, farro, whole wheat pasta, couscous, bulgur, or whole grain bread.

- Healthy Fats: Including sources of healthy fats in your dinner adds richness, flavor, and satiety while supporting brain health and nutrient absorption. Add avocado slices, nuts, seeds, olive oil, coconut oil, or tahini to your salads, grains, vegetables, or protein dishes.

- Flavor Enhancers: Elevate the flavor of your dinner with herbs, spices, condiments, and sauces. Experiment with different combinations of herbs like basil, cilantro, parsley, and mint, as well as spices like garlic, ginger, cumin, paprika, and turmeric. Use condiments like soy sauce, balsamic glaze, salsa, pesto, or tzatziki to add depth and complexity to your meals.

2. Dinner Recipes:

- Grilled Proteins:

- Grilled chicken breasts marinated in lemon, garlic, and herbs, served with roasted vegetables (asparagus, bell peppers, cherry tomatoes) and quinoa pilaf.

- Grilled salmon fillets seasoned with smoked paprika and served with sautéed spinach, mashed sweet potatoes, and a side of mango avocado salsa.

- Grilled tofu skewers with a spicy peanut sauce, served with coconut jasmine rice, stir-fried vegetables (bok choy, bell peppers, snap peas), and a sprinkle of sesame seeds.

- One-Pot Meals:

- Chicken and vegetable stir-fry made with diced chicken breast, broccoli, carrots, bell peppers, snap peas, and cashews, tossed in a homemade teriyaki sauce and served over brown rice or noodles.

- Lentil and vegetable curry simmered with coconut milk, tomatoes, onions, garlic, ginger, and a blend of spices (cumin, coriander, turmeric, curry powder), served with basmati rice and naan bread.

- One-pan baked fish with Mediterranean vegetables (zucchini, eggplant, tomatoes, olives, onions) and a sprinkle of feta cheese, drizzled with olive oil and balsamic glaze.

- Sheet Pan Dinners:

- Sheet pan chicken fajitas with sliced chicken breast, bell peppers, onions, and spices (chili powder, cumin, paprika), served with warm tortillas, guacamole, salsa, and black beans.

- Roasted vegetable and chickpea Buddha bowls with roasted sweet potatoes, cauliflower, Brussels sprouts, chickpeas, and tahini dressing, served over quinoa or couscous.

- Sheet pan shrimp and vegetable skewers with cherry tomatoes, bell peppers, onions, and pineapple chunks, served with coconut rice and a sweet chili glaze.

- Comforting Casseroles:

- Turkey and vegetable shepherd's pie made with ground turkey, mixed vegetables, tomato sauce, and mashed sweet potatoes, baked until golden and bubbly.

- Quinoa and black bean enchilada casserole layered with quinoa, black beans, corn, salsa, and cheese, baked until melted and served with avocado slices and cilantro.

- Mediterranean stuffed peppers filled with ground lamb or beef, quinoa, tomatoes, olives, feta cheese, and fresh herbs, baked until tender and served with a side of Greek yogurt tzatziki sauce.

- Slow Cooker and Instant Pot Meals:

- Slow cooker chicken tikka masala with chicken thighs, tomatoes, onions, garlic, ginger, and a blend of spices (garam masala, turmeric, paprika), served with basmati rice and naan bread.

- Instant Pot lentil soup with green lentils, carrots, celery, onions, garlic, tomatoes, and spinach, seasoned with Italian herbs and served with crusty bread or crackers.

- Slow cooker pork carnitas made with pork shoulder, citrus juice, garlic, onion, and spices (cumin, chili powder, oregano), served in tacos or burrito bowls with your favorite toppings.

- Plant-Based Options:

- Vegan chickpea and vegetable curry with chickpeas, cauliflower, carrots, tomatoes, onions, and coconut milk, seasoned with curry spices and served over rice or quinoa.

- Tofu and vegetable stir-fry with tofu cubes, broccoli, bell peppers, snap peas, and water chestnuts, stir-fried in a savory sauce and served with brown rice or noodles.

- Vegan stuffed portobello mushrooms filled with quinoa, spinach, sun-dried tomatoes, pine nuts, and vegan cheese, baked until tender and served with a side salad.

3. Customization and Variation:

- Customize dinner recipes to suit your taste preferences, dietary needs, and ingredient availability. Feel free to swap out proteins, vegetables, grains, and flavorings to create new and exciting dishes.

- Get creative with seasonings, sauces, and toppings to add variety and flavor to your meals. Don't be afraid to experiment with different herbs, spices, condiments, and garnishes to elevate your dinner creations.

- Use leftovers, pantry staples, and meal prep ingredients to streamline the cooking process and save time in the kitchen.

4. Portion Control and Mindful Eating:

- Pay attention to portion sizes and serving sizes to avoid overeating and support weight management and digestion.

- Eat slowly, savoring each bite, and listen to your body's hunger and fullness cues to guide your eating patterns.

- Practice mindful eating by focusing on the sensory experience of enjoying your dinner, such as the aroma, taste, texture, and appearance of your meal.

5. Hydration and Beverage Choices:

- Pair your dinner with a refreshing beverage like water, herbal tea, or unsweetened iced tea to stay hydrated and support digestion.

- Limit your intake of sugary drinks, sodas, and alcoholic beverages, which can add unnecessary calories and contribute to dehydration and fatigue.

In summary, dinner is an opportunity to nourish your body with a balanced and satisfying meal that includes a variety of nutrient-dense ingredients. By choosing recipes that feature lean proteins, colorful vegetables, whole grains, and healthy fats, you can create delicious and nourishing dinners that support your health and well-being. Experiment with different flavors, cuisines, and cooking techniques to keep your dinner routine exciting and enjoyable, and don't forget to prioritize portion control, mindful eating, and hydration for optimal health and wellness.

Snack Suggestions

Snacks play an important role in maintaining energy levels, preventing hunger between meals, and providing essential nutrients throughout the day. However, choosing nutritious snacks can sometimes be challenging, especially with so many options available. Whether you're looking for something quick and convenient to grab on the go or a satisfying treat to enjoy during a break, here's a comprehensive guide to snack suggestions that are both delicious and nourishing:

1. Components of a Balanced Snack:

- Protein: Including a source of protein in your snack helps promote satiety, stabilize blood sugar levels, and support muscle repair and growth. Choose options such as Greek yogurt, cottage cheese, hard-boiled eggs, turkey slices, tofu, edamame, or nuts and seeds.

- Carbohydrates: Pairing protein with complex carbohydrates provides sustained energy and helps keep you feeling full and satisfied until your next meal. Opt for options like whole fruits, vegetables, whole grain crackers or bread, rice cakes, popcorn, or whole grain tortilla chips.

- Healthy Fats: Adding sources of healthy fats to your snack enhances flavor, satiety, and nutrient absorption. Incorporate options like avocado slices, nut butter, nuts, seeds, olives, or hummus for a satisfying and nutritious snack.

- Fiber: Choosing fiber-rich snacks helps support digestive health, promote feelings of fullness, and regulate blood sugar levels. Include options like raw vegetables, fruit with the skin on, whole grains, nuts, seeds, or legumes for added fiber content.

2. Snack Ideas:

  - Fruit and Nut Combos:

   - Apple slices with almond butter or peanut butter.

- Banana slices topped with Greek yogurt and a sprinkle of granola.

- Celery sticks filled with cream cheese or peanut butter and topped with raisins (ants on a log).

- Sliced pear with ricotta cheese and a drizzle of honey.

- Berries mixed with cottage cheese and a sprinkle of chopped nuts.

- Vegetable Snacks:

- Baby carrots, cucumber slices, and bell pepper strips served with hummus or guacamole.

- Cherry tomatoes stuffed with mozzarella cheese and basil leaves.

- Snap peas dipped in Greek yogurt mixed with ranch seasoning.

- Steamed edamame sprinkled with sea salt and sesame seeds.

- Roasted cauliflower florets tossed in olive oil and garlic powder.

- Dairy-Based Snacks:

- String cheese or cheese cubes paired with whole grain crackers or apple slices.

- Greek yogurt topped with granola, berries, and a drizzle of honey.

- Cottage cheese with pineapple chunks and a sprinkle of cinnamon.

- Hard-boiled eggs sprinkled with paprika and served with cucumber slices.

- Mini caprese skewers with cherry tomatoes, mozzarella balls, and basil leaves.

- Grain-Based Snacks:

- Whole grain crackers topped with hummus, sliced cucumber, and smoked salmon.

- Rice cakes spread with avocado and topped with sliced tomato and cracked black pepper.

- Popcorn seasoned with nutritional yeast, garlic powder, and dried herbs.

- Whole grain pita bread cut into triangles and served with tzatziki sauce.

- Whole wheat tortilla chips with salsa, guacamole, or black bean dip.

- Nut and Seed Snacks:

- Mixed nuts and dried fruit trail mix (almonds, cashews, walnuts, pumpkin seeds, dried cranberries).

- Rice cakes spread with almond butter and sprinkled with chia seeds.

- Toasted coconut chips sprinkled with sea salt.

- Roasted chickpeas seasoned with curry powder and cumin.

- Sunflower seed butter spread on whole grain toast and topped with banana slices.

- **Snack Bars and Bites**:

- Homemade energy bars made with oats, nuts, seeds, dried fruit, and honey or maple syrup.

- Protein bars made with whey protein, nuts, seeds, and dark chocolate chips.

- Date and nut balls rolled in shredded coconut or cocoa powder.

- Granola bars with whole grains, nuts, seeds, and dried fruit.

- Rice crispy treats made with brown rice cereal, almond butter, and honey.

- Smoothies and Smoothie Bowls:

- Protein smoothie made with protein powder, spinach, banana, almond milk, and nut butter.

- Berry smoothie bowl topped with granola, sliced almonds, and shredded coconut.

- Green smoothie with kale, pineapple, mango, coconut water, and chia seeds.

- Chocolate avocado smoothie made with avocado, cocoa powder, banana, Greek yogurt, and almond milk.

- Tropical smoothie bowl with mango, pineapple, coconut milk, spinach, and protein powder.

3. Customization and Variation:

- Get creative with snack combinations by mixing and matching different ingredients and flavors to suit your taste preferences and dietary needs.

- Experiment with different textures, colors, and flavor profiles to keep your snacks interesting and enjoyable.

- Consider batch preparing or meal prepping snacks in advance to have them readily available for busy days or on-the-go snacking.

4. Portion Control and Mindful Eating:

- Pay attention to portion sizes and serving sizes to avoid overeating and support weight management and digestion.

- Practice mindful eating by savoring each bite, chewing slowly, and paying attention to hunger and fullness cues.

- Avoid mindless snacking while distracted by screens or other activities, and instead focus on the sensory experience of enjoying your snack.

5. Hydration and Beverage Choices:

- Pair your snack with a glass of water, herbal tea, or infused water to stay hydrated and support digestion.

- Limit your intake of sugary drinks, sodas, and alcoholic beverages, which can add unnecessary calories and contribute to dehydration and fatigue.

In summary, snacks are an important part of a balanced diet and can provide essential nutrients and energy to fuel your body throughout the day. By choosing nutritious snack options that include a mix of protein, carbohydrates, healthy fats, and fiber, you can support your health and well-being while satisfying your hunger and cravings. Experiment with different snack ideas, flavors, and textures to find what works best for you, and don't forget to prioritize portion control, mindful eating, and hydration for optimal health and wellness.

Chapter 6:

Carbs	Proteins	Fats
• quinoa	• greek yogurt	• avocado
• spinach	• chicken breast	• chia seeds
• kale	• lean beef	• almonds
• berries	• salmon/ fish	• cashews
• apples	• shrimp	• walnuts
• lentils	• turkey	• pecans
• almond/ oat milk	• collagen	• olive oil
• potatoes	• cottage cheese	• cheese
• chickpeas	• whole milk	• pumpkin seeds
• green beans	• eggs	• coconut flour/ oil
• beans	• tuna	

Incorporating Fat-Burning Foods into Your Lifestyle

Incorporating fat-burning foods into your lifestyle can be an effective strategy for supporting weight management, boosting metabolism, and improving overall health and well-being. Fat-burning foods are typically nutrient-dense, low in calories, and contain compounds that promote fat loss, increase metabolism, and enhance satiety. By including these foods in your diet regularly and incorporating them into balanced meals and

202

snacks, you can optimize your body's ability to burn fat and achieve your health and fitness goals. Here's a comprehensive guide to incorporating fat-burning foods into your lifestyle:

1. Understanding Fat-Burning Foods:

- Fat-burning foods are often low in calories and high in nutrients, which means they provide essential vitamins, minerals, and antioxidants while supporting weight loss and metabolism.

- These foods typically contain compounds that boost metabolism, increase thermogenesis (the process of heat production in the body), and enhance fat oxidation (the breakdown of fat for energy).

- Some fat-burning foods also have a high thermic effect, meaning they require more energy to digest, resulting in a greater calorie burn.

- Incorporating a variety of fat-burning foods into your diet can help create a calorie deficit, which is essential for weight loss and fat burning.

2. Key Fat-Burning Nutrients:

- Protein: Protein-rich foods help increase metabolism, promote feelings of fullness, and support muscle growth and repair. Include lean sources of protein such as poultry, fish, tofu, tempeh, legumes, and low-fat dairy in your meals and snacks.

- Fiber: High-fiber foods help regulate appetite, stabilize blood sugar levels, and promote digestive health. Choose fiber-rich foods like fruits, vegetables, whole grains, legumes, nuts, and seeds to support weight loss and fat burning.

- Healthy Fats: Incorporating sources of healthy fats into your diet can help improve satiety, support hormone production, and enhance nutrient absorption. Include foods like avocado, nuts, seeds, olive oil, coconut oil, and fatty fish in your meals and snacks.

- Thermogenic Compounds: Certain foods contain compounds that increase metabolism and promote fat burning. Examples include capsaicin in chili peppers, catechins in green tea, caffeine in coffee, EGCG in matcha tea, and piperine in black pepper.

- Water: Staying hydrated is essential for optimal metabolism and fat burning. Drinking water throughout the day helps support digestion, regulate body temperature, and flush out toxins, all of which contribute to a healthy metabolism.

3. Incorporating Fat-Burning Foods into Your Diet:

- Start by focusing on whole, minimally processed foods that are naturally rich in nutrients and low in added sugars, unhealthy fats, and refined carbohydrates.

- Build meals around lean proteins, fiber-rich vegetables, healthy fats, and complex carbohydrates to create balanced and satisfying dishes that support fat burning.

- Experiment with different cooking methods, flavors, and recipes to keep meals interesting and enjoyable while incorporating fat-burning ingredients.

- Be mindful of portion sizes and avoid overeating, even with healthy foods. Remember that excess calories, regardless of the source, can hinder weight loss and fat burning.

- Plan and prepare meals and snacks in advance to ensure you have nutritious options readily available when hunger strikes. This can help prevent impulsive choices and overeating unhealthy foods.

- Incorporate fat-burning foods into every meal and snack throughout the day to keep your metabolism revved up and support consistent fat burning.

- Be patient and consistent with your dietary changes, as sustainable weight loss and fat burning take time and effort. Focus on making gradual, long-term lifestyle changes rather than seeking quick fixes or extreme measures.

4. Examples of Fat-Burning Foods:

- Lean Proteins: Chicken breast, turkey breast, fish (salmon, tuna, trout), tofu, tempeh, lean beef, eggs, Greek yogurt, cottage cheese.

- Fiber-Rich Vegetables: Leafy greens (spinach, kale, Swiss chard), cruciferous vegetables (broccoli, cauliflower, Brussels sprouts), bell peppers, cucumber, zucchini, celery, carrots.

- Whole Grains: Quinoa, brown rice, oats, barley, bulgur, whole wheat bread, whole grain pasta, farro, buckwheat.

- Healthy Fats: Avocado, nuts (almonds, walnuts, pistachios), seeds (chia seeds, flaxseeds, pumpkin seeds), olive oil, coconut oil, fatty fish (salmon, mackerel, sardines).

- Thermogenic Foods: Chili peppers, green tea, coffee, matcha tea, ginger, garlic, cinnamon, black pepper, turmeric.

- Hydrating Foods: Water-rich fruits (watermelon, berries, citrus fruits), vegetables (cucumber, celery, tomatoes), herbal teas, coconut water.

5. Meal Planning and Preparation:

- Plan meals and snacks ahead of time to ensure you have a variety of fat-burning foods on hand.

- Batch cook ingredients like grilled chicken, roasted vegetables, quinoa, and beans to use in multiple meals throughout the week.

- Prep grab-and-go snacks like sliced veggies with hummus, Greek yogurt with berries, or homemade trail mix to have healthy options available when hunger strikes.

- Use portion control tools like measuring cups, food scales, and portioned containers to help you manage serving sizes and avoid overeating.

6. Balanced Lifestyle Habits:

- In addition to incorporating fat-burning foods into your diet, prioritize other aspects of a healthy lifestyle such as regular physical activity, adequate sleep, stress management, and hydration.

- Aim for a combination of cardiovascular exercise, strength training, and flexibility exercises to maximize calorie burn, build lean muscle mass, and support overall health and fitness.

- Practice stress-reducing activities like yoga, meditation, deep breathing exercises, or spending time in nature to lower cortisol levels and reduce stress-induced cravings for unhealthy foods.

- Get sufficient sleep each night, as lack of sleep can disrupt hormone balance, increase appetite, and hinder weight loss efforts.

- Stay hydrated by drinking plenty of water throughout the day, as dehydration can negatively impact metabolism and energy levels.

In summary, incorporating fat-burning foods into your lifestyle involves choosing nutrient-dense, metabolism-boosting ingredients that support weight loss and overall health. By focusing on lean proteins, fiber-rich vegetables, healthy fats, and thermogenic compounds, you can create balanced meals and snacks that optimize your body's ability to burn fat and achieve your health and fitness goals. Be mindful of portion sizes, plan and prepare meals ahead of time, and prioritize other aspects of a healthy lifestyle to support long-term success. With consistency, patience, and dedication, you can embrace a lifestyle that promotes fat burning, enhances metabolism, and fosters overall well-being.

Grocery Shopping Tips

Grocery shopping is a fundamental aspect of maintaining a healthy and balanced diet. Making informed choices at the grocery store can help you stock up on nutritious foods while staying within your budget. Here are some extensive and comprehensive grocery shopping tips to help you make the most out of your shopping trips:

1. Plan Ahead:

- Before heading to the grocery store, take some time to plan your meals for the week. Consider your schedule, dietary preferences, and any special occasions or events.

- Make a list of the ingredients you'll need for each meal, as well as any staples or household items you're running low on.

- Check your pantry, refrigerator, and freezer to see what ingredients you already have on hand to avoid buying duplicates.

- Consider incorporating seasonal produce and sales or promotions into your meal planning to save money and enjoy fresh, in-season ingredients.

2. Stick to a Budget:

- Set a budget for your grocery shopping trip and try to stick to it. Consider using cash or a debit card rather than credit cards to help you stay within your budget.

- Compare prices and look for sales, discounts, and coupons to maximize your savings. Be mindful of unit prices to ensure you're getting the best value for your money.

- Consider shopping at discount stores, farmers' markets, or buying in bulk for additional savings on groceries.

3. Choose Nutrient-Dense Foods:

- Focus on filling your cart with nutrient-dense foods that provide essential vitamins, minerals, and antioxidants. These include fruits, vegetables, whole grains, lean proteins, and healthy fats.

- Prioritize fresh, whole foods over processed or packaged items whenever possible. Look for minimally processed options with short ingredient lists and avoid products with added sugars, unhealthy fats, and artificial additives.

- Opt for a variety of colorful fruits and vegetables to ensure you're getting a wide range of nutrients and phytochemicals. Choose whole grains like brown rice, quinoa, oats, and whole wheat bread or pasta for fiber and complex carbohydrates.

- Select lean proteins such as chicken, turkey, fish, tofu, tempeh, beans, and legumes to support muscle repair and growth, as well as overall health and satiety.

- Include sources of healthy fats like avocado, nuts, seeds, olive oil, and fatty fish to promote heart health, brain function, and nutrient absorption.

4. Read Labels Carefully:

- Take the time to read food labels and ingredient lists to make informed choices about the products you're purchasing.

- Pay attention to serving sizes, calorie counts, and nutrient content per serving to ensure you're meeting your dietary needs and goals.

- Look for foods that are low in added sugars, unhealthy fats, sodium, and artificial additives. Choose products with recognizable ingredients and avoid highly processed or refined foods.

5. Shop the Perimeter:

- When navigating the grocery store, focus on shopping the perimeter where fresh produce, meat, dairy, and whole foods are typically located.

- Fill your cart with a variety of fruits and vegetables, lean proteins, dairy or dairy alternatives, and whole grains from these outer aisles.

- Limit your time in the inner aisles where processed and packaged foods, snacks, and sugary beverages are often found. If you do venture into these aisles, stick to your list and avoid impulse purchases.

6. Be Flexible and Open-Minded:

- Be open to trying new foods, flavors, and recipes to keep your meals interesting and enjoyable.

- Take advantage of the variety of options available at the grocery store, including ethnic foods, specialty products, and seasonal produce.

- Don't be afraid to experiment with different cooking techniques, ingredients, and cuisines to expand your culinary repertoire and discover new favorites.

7. Practice Safe and Sustainable Shopping:

- Choose environmentally friendly and sustainable options whenever possible, such as organic, locally sourced, and ethically produced foods.

- Bring reusable shopping bags, produce bags, and containers to reduce waste and minimize your environmental impact.

- Check for signs of freshness and quality when selecting fruits, vegetables, meat, and seafood. Choose items with vibrant colors, firm textures, and pleasant smells to ensure they're fresh and ripe.

8. Stay Organized and Efficient:

- Organize your shopping list by categories (e.g., produce, dairy, pantry staples) to streamline your shopping trip and save time in the store.

- Start with perishable items like produce, meat, and dairy, and finish with non-perishable items like grains, canned goods, and household items.

- Avoid shopping when you're hungry, as this can lead to impulse purchases and unhealthy food choices. Instead, eat a balanced meal or snack before heading to the grocery store to help you make more mindful decisions.

- Consider using grocery shopping apps or online grocery delivery services for added convenience and flexibility, especially if you have a busy schedule or limited mobility.

By following these comprehensive grocery shopping tips, you can make informed choices at the grocery store, stock up on nutritious foods, and stay within your budget. With careful planning, organization, and a focus on nutrient-dense options, you can support your health and well-being while enjoying delicious and satisfying meals at home.

Cooking Techniques

Cooking techniques encompass a wide range of methods used to prepare and cook food, each with its unique principles, applications, and effects on the flavor, texture, and nutritional content of the ingredients. Mastering various cooking techniques allows home cooks and professional chefs alike to create delicious, well-balanced meals that showcase the natural flavors of the ingredients while achieving desired results in terms of taste, appearance, and consistency. Here's an extensive and comprehensive overview of some common cooking techniques:

1. Sautéing:

- Sautéing involves cooking food quickly in a small amount of oil or fat over medium to high heat in a shallow pan.

- This technique is commonly used for vegetables, proteins (such as chicken, fish, or tofu), and aromatics like garlic and onions.

- To sauté effectively, ensure the pan is hot before adding ingredients, and use a high smoke point oil like olive oil or grapeseed oil.

- Constantly move the ingredients around the pan with a spatula or wooden spoon to prevent sticking and ensure even cooking.

2. Stir-Frying:

- Stir-frying is similar to sautéing but typically involves higher heat and constant stirring of ingredients in a wok or large skillet.

- This technique is commonly used in Asian cuisine and is ideal for quickly cooking thinly sliced vegetables, meat, and seafood.

- Ingredients are cooked in a small amount of oil over high heat, with frequent tossing and stirring to ensure even cooking and to prevent burning.

3. Grilling:

- Grilling involves cooking food over an open flame or hot grill grate, imparting a smoky flavor and attractive grill marks.

- This technique is ideal for cooking meats, poultry, seafood, vegetables, and even fruits.

- To grill effectively, preheat the grill to the desired temperature, oil the grate to prevent sticking, and monitor the cooking process closely to prevent burning.

- Grilling can be done using direct heat (placing food directly over the flame or heat source) or indirect heat (placing food to the side of the heat source), depending on the type of food being cooked and desired results.

4. Roasting:

- Roasting involves cooking food in an oven at high heat, typically between 350°F to 450°F (175°C to 230°C).

- This technique is commonly used for meats, poultry, vegetables, and root crops, resulting in caramelization, browning, and rich flavors.

- To roast effectively, arrange food in a single layer on a baking sheet or roasting pan, season as desired, and roast until golden brown and tender, turning occasionally for even cooking.

5. Baking:

- Baking involves cooking food in an enclosed oven using dry heat, typically at temperatures ranging from 300°F to 450°F (150°C to 230°C).

- This technique is commonly used for bread, cakes, cookies, pastries, and casseroles.

- Baking relies on the chemical reactions between ingredients such as flour, sugar, eggs, and leavening agents (such as baking powder or yeast) to produce light, airy textures and delicious flavors.

6. Boiling:

- Boiling involves cooking food in a liquid, typically water or broth, at or near its boiling point (212°F or 100°C at sea level).

- This technique is commonly used for pasta, grains, beans, vegetables, and eggs.

- Boiling cooks food quickly and evenly, but prolonged boiling can lead to nutrient loss and flavor dilution. To prevent overcooking, it's essential to monitor the cooking time and remove food from the liquid promptly when done.

7. Steaming:

- Steaming involves cooking food by exposing it to steam vapor in a covered vessel, such as a steamer basket, bamboo steamer, or microwave steamer.

- This technique is ideal for preserving the natural flavors, colors, and nutrients of ingredients, especially vegetables, fish, poultry, and dumplings.

- Steaming cooks food gently and evenly, resulting in tender textures and vibrant colors, without the need for added fats or oils.

8. Braising:

- Braising involves cooking food slowly in a small amount of liquid, typically broth, wine, or tomato sauce, in a covered pot or Dutch oven.

- This technique is ideal for tougher cuts of meat, poultry, and root vegetables, resulting in tender, flavorful dishes.

- Braising combines dry heat cooking (searing or browning) with moist heat cooking (simmering or stewing) to break down tough connective tissues and infuse the ingredients with rich, savory flavors.

9. Frying:

- Frying involves cooking food by submerging it in hot oil or fat, resulting in crispy exteriors and tender interiors.

- This technique can be categorized into shallow frying (cooking food partially submerged in oil) and deep frying (cooking food fully submerged in oil).

- While deep frying is known for producing indulgent, crispy foods like French fries, chicken wings, and doughnuts, shallow frying is used for pan-frying items like fish fillets, schnitzel, and eggplant slices.

10. Poaching:

- Poaching involves cooking food gently in simmering liquid, such as water, broth, or wine, until tender and fully cooked.

- This technique is commonly used for delicate proteins like fish, chicken, eggs, and fruit.

- Poaching helps preserve the natural flavors and textures of ingredients while adding subtle flavors from the cooking liquid and aromatics like herbs, spices, and citrus zest.

11. Broiling:

- Broiling involves cooking food under direct heat in the oven, similar to grilling but with the heat source located above the food.

- This technique is ideal for quickly cooking meats, poultry, seafood, and vegetables, resulting in caramelization and browning on the surface.

- To broil effectively, preheat the broiler, arrange food on a broiler pan or baking sheet, and place it on the top oven rack closest to the heating element. Monitor the cooking process closely to prevent burning.

12. Smoking:

- Smoking involves cooking food slowly and gently over low heat in a smoker or grill, using wood chips or chunks to produce smoke.

- This technique infuses food with rich, smoky flavors and tenderizes tough cuts of meat, poultry, and fish.

- Smoking can be done using hot smoking (cooking food directly over heat) or cold smoking (exposing food to smoke without direct heat), depending on the desired results and the type of food being smoked.

13. Sous Vide:

- Sous vide involves cooking food in vacuum-sealed bags submerged in a water bath at precise temperatures using an immersion circulator.

- This technique allows for precise temperature control and even cooking, resulting in perfectly cooked proteins, vegetables, and desserts with minimal loss of moisture and nutrients.

- Sous vide cooking requires longer cooking times compared to traditional methods but produces consistently tender, flavorful dishes.

14. Blanching:

- Blanching involves briefly cooking food in boiling water, then quickly transferring it to an ice bath to stop the cooking process.

- This technique is commonly used to partially cook vegetables before freezing or to remove skins from fruits and vegetables.

- Blanching helps preserve the color, texture, and flavor of ingredients while also reducing microbial contamination and enzymatic activity.

15. Fermentation:

- Fermentation involves the transformation of food by beneficial bacteria, yeast, or fungi, resulting in unique flavors, textures, and nutritional profiles.

- This technique is used to produce foods like yogurt, cheese, sourdough bread, kimchi, sauerkraut, kombucha, and pickles.

- Fermentation enhances the digestibility, shelf-life, and probiotic content of foods while also imparting tangy, complex flavors.

16. Curing:

- Curing involves preserving food by soaking it in a salt solution or dry-rubbing it with salt and other seasonings, then allowing it to air dry or age.

- This technique is used to produce cured meats like bacon, ham, salami, and prosciutto, as well as cured fish like gravlax and smoked salmon.

- Curing imparts flavor, extends shelf-life, and inhibits bacterial growth, resulting in savory, complex products with a characteristic salty taste.

17. Deglazing:

- Deglazing involves adding liquid (such as wine, broth, or vinegar) to a hot pan to loosen and dissolve browned bits of food stuck to the bottom, known as fond.

- This technique is used to create flavorful sauces and gravies to accompany meat, poultry, and fish dishes.

- Deglazing also helps incorporate the flavors of aromatics like onions, garlic, and herbs into the sauce while adding depth and complexity.

18. Emulsifying:

- Emulsifying involves combining two immiscible liquids, such as oil and water, into a stable mixture by dispersing one phase into the other using an emulsifier.

- This technique is used to create creamy, smooth sauces like vinaigrettes, mayonnaise, hollandaise, and béarnaise.

- Emulsifiers like egg yolks, mustard, and lecithin help bind the oil and water molecules together, preventing separation and ensuring a uniform consistency.

19. Reduction:

- Reduction involves simmering a liquid, such as stock, wine, or vinegar, over low heat to evaporate water and concentrate flavors.

- This technique is used to create rich, flavorful sauces, glazes, and syrups with a thick, glossy consistency.

- Reduction intensifies the natural flavors of ingredients and creates a complex, nuanced sauce or reduction that can elevate a dish.

20. Tempering:

- Tempering involves slowly raising the temperature of a delicate ingredient, such as eggs or chocolate, by gradually adding a hot liquid or melted fat.

- This technique is used to prevent curdling, seizing, or overheating, ensuring smooth, creamy textures and glossy finishes.

- Tempering is commonly used in recipes for custards, sauces, ganache, and chocolate confections to achieve the desired consistency and appearance.

21. Infusing:

- Infusing involves steeping ingredients like herbs, spices, citrus zest, or aromatics in a liquid (such as oil, vinegar, or alcohol) to impart flavor.

- This technique is used to add depth and complexity to sauces, dressings, marinades, syrups, and beverages.

- Infusing allows the flavors of the ingredients to meld together over time, resulting in infused liquids with rich, aromatic profiles.

22. Whipping:

- Whipping involves incorporating air into a mixture, typically through vigorous beating or whisking, to increase volume and create light, fluffy textures.

- This technique is commonly used to whip cream, egg whites, and butter to stiff peaks for desserts like mousse, soufflés, and frostings.

- Whipping aerates the mixture, trapping air bubbles that expand during baking or chilling, resulting in airy, tender finished products.

23. Macerating:

- Macerating involves soaking fruit, berries, or dried fruits in a liquid (such as sugar, alcohol, or citrus juice) to soften, sweeten, and enhance their flavor.

- This technique is used to create fruit compotes, preserves, jams, and dessert toppings, as well as flavored liqueurs and infusions.

- Macerating extracts natural juices from the fruit while infusing it with the flavors of the macerating liquid, resulting in tender, flavorful fruit preparations.

24. Chilling and Freezing:

- Chilling and freezing involve lowering the temperature of food to preserve freshness, slow microbial growth, and extend shelf-life.

- This technique is used to store perishable items like meat, poultry, seafood, dairy products, and prepared meals.

- Chilling and freezing help maintain the quality, texture, and flavor of ingredients while also preventing food waste and allowing for convenient meal preparation and storage.

25. Reheating and Reviving:

- Reheating and reviving involve gently warming or refreshing cooked or leftover food to restore its temperature, texture, and flavor.

- This technique is used to reheat chilled or frozen foods, revive stale bread or pastries, and refresh wilted or limp vegetables.

- Reheating and reviving can be done using various methods such as stovetop heating, oven baking, microwave reheating, or steaming, depending on the type of food and desired results.

26. Combination Cooking:

- Combination cooking involves combining two or more cooking techniques to achieve optimal results, such as searing followed by braising or roasting followed by broiling.

- This technique allows for greater control over the cooking process and can result in dishes with complex flavors, textures, and appearances.

- Combination cooking is commonly used in recipes for stews, casseroles, roasts, and grilled or roasted meats and vegetables to enhance flavor and tenderness while achieving caramelization, browning, or crispiness.

By mastering these various cooking techniques and understanding their applications, home cooks and chefs can elevate their culinary skills and create delicious, well-balanced meals that showcase the natural flavors of the ingredients. Experimenting with different methods, recipes, and ingredients allows for endless creativity and innovation in the kitchen, making cooking an enjoyable and rewarding experience for cooks of all levels.

Dining Out Strategies

Dining out can be a fun and enjoyable experience, but it can also present challenges when trying to make healthy choices and stay on track with your dietary goals. However, with some planning and smart strategies, you can enjoy eating out while still making nutritious choices that support your health and well-being. Here are extensive and comprehensive dining out strategies to help you navigate restaurants and make healthier choices:

1. Research Restaurants in Advance:

- Before heading out to eat, take some time to research restaurants in your area that offer healthy options.

- Look for restaurants that prioritize fresh, whole ingredients, offer customizable dishes, and provide nutritional information on their menus.

- Check online reviews, menus, and social media accounts for insights into the restaurant's atmosphere, menu options, and customer experiences.

2. Review the Menu Carefully:

- Once you arrive at the restaurant, take a few moments to review the menu carefully before making your selection.

- Look for dishes that are grilled, baked, steamed, or roasted rather than fried or sautéed in heavy sauces or oils.

- Choose dishes that feature lean proteins, whole grains, and plenty of vegetables, and consider asking for modifications or substitutions to customize your meal to your preferences.

- Pay attention to portion sizes and consider sharing an entree or ordering a smaller portion to avoid overeating.

3. Balance Your Plate:

- Aim to create a balanced meal that includes a variety of nutrient-dense foods from different food groups.

- Start with a salad or vegetable-based appetizer to help fill up on fiber and nutrients before the main course.

- Include lean proteins like grilled chicken, fish, tofu, or legumes, along with whole grains like brown rice, quinoa, or whole wheat pasta.

- Incorporate plenty of vegetables into your meal, whether as side dishes, toppings, or main components of the dish.

- Limit or avoid high-calorie and high-fat items like fried foods, creamy sauces, and excessive amounts of cheese or butter.

4. Ask Questions and Make Requests:

- Don't be afraid to ask your server questions about menu items, ingredients, and preparation methods.

- Inquire about how dishes are cooked, whether they contain any hidden ingredients or allergens, and if modifications or substitutions are possible.

- Request dressings, sauces, and condiments on the side so you can control the amount you use, and ask for steamed or lightly seasoned vegetables instead of heavy sides like fries or mashed potatoes.

- Be polite and respectful when making requests, and tip generously for good service.

5. Practice Portion Control:

- Be mindful of portion sizes, which can often be larger than necessary when dining out.

- Consider sharing an appetizer, entree, or dessert with a dining companion to reduce the amount of food you consume.

- Ask for a to-go container when your meal arrives and portion out a suitable amount of food to take home for another meal.

- Listen to your body's hunger and fullness cues and stop eating when you feel satisfied, rather than finishing everything on your plate out of habit.

6. Be Mindful of Beverages:

- Be mindful of your beverage choices, as sugary drinks, alcoholic beverages, and calorie-laden cocktails can contribute to excess calorie intake.

- Opt for water, sparkling water, unsweetened tea, or black coffee as healthier drink options that won't add extra calories.

- If you choose to indulge in alcoholic beverages, do so in moderation and consider lower-calorie options like light beer, wine spritzers, or mixed drinks made with soda water and fresh citrus juice.

7. Enjoy Mindfully:

- Practice mindful eating by slowing down, savoring each bite, and paying attention to the flavors, textures, and sensations of the food.

- Put your fork down between bites, chew your food thoroughly, and engage in conversation with your dining companions to enhance the dining experience.

- Avoid distractions like smartphones, television, or work-related tasks, and focus on enjoying the meal and the company you're with.

- Be forgiving of yourself if you indulge in a less-than-healthy choice and remember that one meal or snack doesn't define your overall eating habits.

8. Plan for Special Occasions:

- For special occasions or celebrations, consider choosing a restaurant that offers healthier options or allows for customization of dishes.

- If you know you'll be dining out for a special occasion, plan ahead by eating lighter meals throughout the day to balance out any indulgences you may enjoy during the celebration.

- Practice moderation and portion control, and allow yourself to enjoy your favorite dishes without guilt or restriction.

9. Listen to Your Body:

- Pay attention to how different foods make you feel physically and emotionally, and make choices that align with your individual preferences and dietary needs.

- Trust your instincts and choose foods that nourish your body and satisfy your cravings, rather than following strict rules or restrictions.

- Practice self-compassion and flexibility, and remember that eating out should be an enjoyable and pleasurable experience that adds to your overall quality of life.

10. Practice Consistency, Not Perfection:

- Aim for consistency in your eating habits rather than striving for perfection when dining out.

- Focus on making balanced choices most of the time, but allow yourself the flexibility to enjoy occasional indulgences or treats without guilt.

- Be patient and kind to yourself, and remember that healthy eating is about progress, not perfection.

By implementing these dining out strategies, you can make healthier choices when eating out while still enjoying delicious meals and socializing with friends and family. With a little planning, mindfulness, and flexibility, you can navigate restaurants and make choices that support your health and well-being without sacrificing flavor or enjoyment.

Chapter 7:

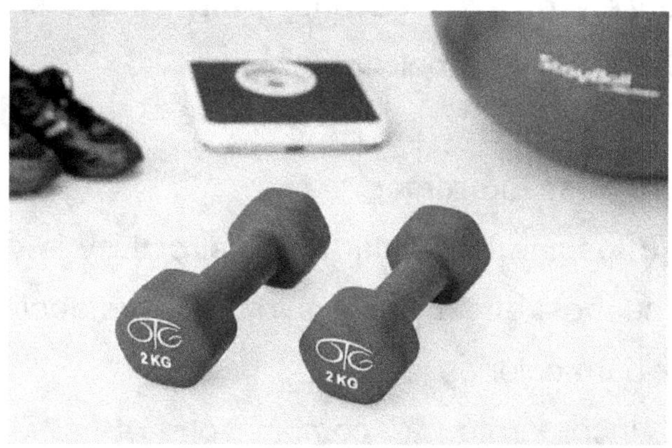

Exercise and Lifestyle Factors for Maximizing Metabolism

Maximizing metabolism involves adopting a holistic approach that incorporates regular physical activity, healthy eating habits, adequate sleep, stress management, and other lifestyle factors that support metabolic health. By combining exercise with lifestyle modifications, you can optimize your metabolism to promote fat burning, improve energy levels, and maintain a healthy weight.

Here's an extensive and comprehensive overview of exercise and lifestyle factors for maximizing metabolism:

1. Regular Exercise:

- Engaging in regular physical activity is one of the most effective ways to boost metabolism and burn calories.

- Incorporate a combination of aerobic exercise, strength training, and flexibility exercises into your weekly routine for optimal results.

- Aerobic exercise, such as walking, jogging, cycling, swimming, or dancing, increases heart rate and calorie expenditure, helping to burn fat and improve cardiovascular health.

- Strength training, using weights, resistance bands, or bodyweight exercises, helps build lean muscle mass, which is more metabolically active than fat tissue and can increase resting metabolic rate.

- Aim for at least 150 minutes of moderate-intensity aerobic exercise or 75 minutes of vigorous-intensity aerobic exercise per week, along with two or more days of strength training exercises targeting major muscle groups.

2. High-Intensity Interval Training (HIIT):

- HIIT involves alternating between short bursts of intense exercise and brief periods of rest or lower-intensity exercise.

- This type of training can increase metabolism and calorie burning both during and after exercise, known as the "afterburn" effect or excess post-exercise oxygen consumption (EPOC).

- Incorporate HIIT workouts into your routine 1-3 times per week, focusing on exercises like sprinting, jumping rope, or bodyweight exercises performed at maximum effort for short intervals followed by periods of recovery.

3. Stay Active Throughout the Day:

- In addition to structured exercise sessions, aim to stay active throughout the day by incorporating more movement into your daily routine.

- Take regular breaks to stand up, stretch, and walk around if you have a sedentary job or lifestyle.

- Use a standing desk, take the stairs instead of the elevator, walk or bike to work, and incorporate physical activity into leisure activities like gardening, dancing, or playing sports.

4. Build Muscle Mass:

- Muscle tissue is metabolically active and requires more energy (calories) to maintain compared to fat tissue.

- Incorporate strength training exercises into your routine to build and maintain lean muscle mass, which can increase resting metabolic rate and improve overall metabolic health.

- Focus on compound exercises that target multiple muscle groups simultaneously, such as squats, lunges, deadlifts, push-ups, and rows.

- Gradually increase the intensity, frequency, and resistance of your strength training workouts over time to continue challenging your muscles and stimulating growth.

5. Eat a Balanced Diet:

- Consuming a balanced diet that includes a variety of nutrient-dense foods is essential for supporting metabolism and overall health.

- Prioritize whole, minimally processed foods like fruits, vegetables, lean proteins, whole grains, and healthy fats.

- Include protein-rich foods in each meal and snack to support muscle repair and growth, as well as to increase satiety and prevent overeating.

- Incorporate complex carbohydrates for sustained energy levels, fiber to aid digestion and promote feelings of fullness, and healthy fats for hormone production and nutrient absorption.

6. Stay Hydrated:

- Drinking an adequate amount of water is essential for optimal metabolic function and overall health.

- Aim to drink at least 8-10 cups of water per day, or more if you're physically active or live in a hot climate.

- Stay hydrated throughout the day by sipping water regularly and incorporating hydrating foods like fruits, vegetables, and soups into your diet.

7. Get Sufficient Sleep:

- Adequate sleep is crucial for regulating metabolism, hormone production, appetite control, and energy levels.

- Aim for 7-9 hours of quality sleep per night, and prioritize establishing a consistent sleep schedule that allows for sufficient rest and recovery.

- Create a relaxing bedtime routine, minimize screen time before bed, and create a comfortable sleep environment to promote restful sleep.

8. Manage Stress Levels:

- Chronic stress can negatively impact metabolism and contribute to weight gain, inflammation, and metabolic dysfunction.

- Practice stress-reduction techniques such as deep breathing, meditation, yoga, tai chi, or progressive muscle relaxation to help manage stress levels and promote relaxation.

- Incorporate regular physical activity, spend time outdoors, prioritize leisure activities, and cultivate social connections to support mental and emotional well-being.

9. Limit Alcohol and Sugary Beverages:

- Limiting alcohol intake and sugary beverages can help reduce empty calories and excess sugar consumption, which can contribute to weight gain and metabolic imbalances.

- Choose water, herbal tea, or sparkling water with lemon or lime as hydrating alternatives to sugary sodas, energy drinks, and alcoholic beverages.

- Enjoy alcohol in moderation and be mindful of portion sizes and calorie content, opting for lower-calorie options like light beer, dry wine, or spirits mixed with soda water and fresh citrus.

10. Practice Mindful Eating:

- Pay attention to hunger and fullness cues, and eat mindfully by slowing down, chewing your food thoroughly, and savoring each bite.

- Avoid distractions while eating, such as watching TV, using electronic devices, or eating on the go, which can lead to overeating and poor digestion.

- Tune into your body's signals of hunger and satiety, and stop eating when you feel comfortably satisfied, rather than continuing to eat out of habit or boredom.

11. Seek Professional Guidance:

- If you're struggling to optimize your metabolism or make sustainable lifestyle changes, consider seeking guidance from a registered dietitian, certified personal trainer, or healthcare professional.

- A professional can provide personalized recommendations, support, and accountability to help you achieve your goals and overcome any barriers or challenges you may encounter along the way.

By incorporating these exercise and lifestyle factors into your daily routine, you can maximize your metabolism, support fat burning, and improve overall health and well-being. Remember that consistency, patience, and self-care are key to long-term success, and focus on making gradual, sustainable changes that align with your individual needs and preferences.

Importance of Physical Activity

Physical activity plays a crucial role in promoting overall health and well-being by positively impacting various aspects of physical, mental, and emotional health. From improving cardiovascular fitness and muscle strength to boosting mood and reducing the risk of chronic diseases, regular physical activity is essential for maintaining a healthy lifestyle. Here's an extensive and comprehensive overview of the importance of physical activity:

1. Enhances Cardiovascular Health:

- Regular physical activity, such as aerobic exercise, helps strengthen the heart muscle, improve circulation, and lower blood pressure.

- Engaging in cardiorespiratory activities like walking, jogging, cycling, swimming, or dancing can reduce the risk of heart disease, stroke, and other cardiovascular conditions.

- Aerobic exercise increases heart rate and breathing rate, improving the efficiency of the cardiovascular system and enhancing overall cardiovascular health.

2. Promotes Weight Management:

- Physical activity plays a key role in energy balance by burning calories and supporting weight management.

- Regular exercise helps increase metabolism, build lean muscle mass, and reduce body fat, leading to improved body composition and weight control.

- Combining aerobic exercise with strength training can optimize calorie burning, muscle growth, and fat loss, contributing to a healthy weight and body mass index (BMI).

3. Strengthens Muscles and Bones:

- Resistance training, such as lifting weights, using resistance bands, or performing bodyweight exercises, helps strengthen muscles and bones.

- Weight-bearing activities like walking, running, and jumping promote bone density and reduce the risk of osteoporosis and fractures, especially in older adults.

- Building and maintaining muscle mass through strength training can improve balance, stability, and functional capacity, reducing the risk of falls and injuries.

4. Improves Mental Health and Well-being:

- Physical activity has profound effects on mental health and emotional well-being by reducing stress, anxiety, and depression.

- Exercise stimulates the release of endorphins, neurotransmitters that promote feelings of happiness and relaxation, leading to improved mood and emotional resilience.

- Regular physical activity can enhance cognitive function, memory, and concentration, as well as reduce the risk of cognitive decline and dementia later in life.

5. Boosts Energy Levels and Vitality:

- Engaging in physical activity increases energy levels, reduces fatigue, and improves overall vitality and quality of life.

- Exercise enhances oxygen delivery and nutrient circulation throughout the body, promoting cellular energy production and metabolic efficiency.

- Regular physical activity can improve sleep quality, increase daytime alertness, and enhance productivity and performance in daily activities.

6. Reduces the Risk of Chronic Diseases:

- Physical activity is associated with a reduced risk of developing chronic diseases such as type 2 diabetes, hypertension, certain cancers, and metabolic syndrome.

- Regular exercise helps control blood sugar levels, improve insulin sensitivity, and reduce inflammation, lowering the risk of insulin resistance and type 2 diabetes.

- Maintaining a physically active lifestyle is linked to a lower incidence of certain cancers, including breast, colon, lung, and prostate cancer, as well as a decreased risk of metabolic syndrome and other metabolic disorders.

7. Supports Longevity and Healthy Aging:

- Regular physical activity is associated with increased longevity and a higher quality of life in older adults.

- Exercise helps preserve mobility, independence, and functional capacity as people age, reducing the risk of disability and chronic health conditions.

- Engaging in physical activity throughout life promotes healthy aging by maintaining muscle mass, bone density, cognitive function, and cardiovascular health.

8. Fosters Social Connections and Community:

- Physical activity provides opportunities for social interaction, camaraderie, and community engagement.

- Joining group fitness classes, sports teams, or outdoor recreational activities allows individuals to connect with others who share similar interests and goals.

- Building social connections through physical activity can enhance motivation, accountability, and enjoyment, leading to greater adherence to exercise routines and long-term sustainability.

9. Improves Self-esteem and Body Image:

- Regular physical activity can boost self-esteem, self-confidence, and body image by promoting feelings of accomplishment, competence, and self-efficacy.

- Achieving fitness goals, improving physical performance, and enhancing body composition through exercise can positively impact how individuals perceive themselves and their bodies.

- Engaging in physical activity that is enjoyable and personally meaningful fosters a positive relationship with exercise and promotes a healthy body image.

10. Sets a Positive Example for Others:

- Leading an active lifestyle sets a positive example for family members, friends, and colleagues, inspiring others to prioritize their own health and well-being.

- Being physically active can influence social norms and cultural attitudes toward exercise, promoting a culture of health, fitness, and vitality within communities.

- Serving as a role model for physical activity encourages others to adopt healthy behaviors and contributes to the collective effort to improve public health and prevent chronic diseases.

In conclusion, physical activity is essential for promoting overall health, vitality, and well-being across the lifespan. From reducing the risk of chronic diseases to enhancing mental health and fostering social connections, regular exercise offers numerous benefits that contribute to a healthier, happier life. By incorporating physical activity into your daily routine and making it a priority, you can maximize your potential for optimal health and longevity.

Strength Training vs. Cardio

Strength training and cardio (aerobic exercise) are two distinct forms of exercise, each offering unique benefits for overall health, fitness, and well-being. While both types of exercise contribute to physical fitness, they target different aspects of fitness and serve complementary roles in a well-rounded exercise program. Here's an extensive and comprehensive comparison of strength training vs. cardio:

Strength Training:

1. Definition and Benefits:

- Strength training, also known as resistance training or weight training, involves performing exercises that challenge the muscles against resistance.

- The primary goal of strength training is to increase muscle strength, power, endurance, and hypertrophy (muscle growth).

- Strength training exercises typically use free weights (dumbbells, barbells), weight machines, resistance bands, or body weight as resistance.

2. Muscle Development:

- Strength training stimulates muscle fibers to adapt and grow stronger in response to resistance, resulting in increased muscle mass, definition, and tone.

- Progressive overload, gradually increasing the resistance or intensity of exercises over time, is key to stimulating muscle growth and strength gains.

3. Metabolic Benefits:

-    Strength training increases resting metabolic rate (RMR) by building lean muscle mass, which requires more calories to maintain compared to fat tissue.

- Muscle tissue is metabolically active, so increasing muscle mass through strength training can help boost metabolism and support weight management.

4. Bone Health:

- Strength training exercises that load the bones, such as weight-bearing and resistance exercises, stimulate bone remodeling and help maintain bone density.

- Regular strength training can reduce the risk of osteoporosis and fractures, especially in older adults, by promoting bone strength and integrity.

5. Functional Strength:

- Strength training improves functional strength, stability, and mobility, enhancing performance in daily activities, sports, and recreational pursuits.

- Compound exercises that target multiple muscle groups simultaneously, such as squats, deadlifts, lunges, and push-ups, promote overall functional fitness and movement proficiency.

6. Injury Prevention:

- Strengthening muscles and connective tissues through resistance training can help prevent injuries by improving joint stability, balance, and coordination.

- Targeting weak or imbalanced muscle groups can correct muscle imbalances and reduce the risk of overuse injuries and musculoskeletal problems.

7. Flexibility and Range of Motion:

- While strength training primarily focuses on building strength and muscle mass, incorporating dynamic stretches and mobility exercises can improve flexibility and range of motion.

- Performing full range-of-motion exercises and incorporating stretching into your strength training routine can enhance joint flexibility and movement quality.

Cardio (Aerobic Exercise):

1. Definition and Benefits:

- Cardiovascular exercise, commonly referred to as cardio or aerobic exercise, involves activities that elevate heart rate and increase oxygen consumption to improve cardiovascular fitness.

- The primary goal of cardio exercise is to enhance heart and lung function, increase endurance, and burn calories for weight management.

2. Heart Health:

- Cardiovascular exercise strengthens the heart muscle, improves circulation, and enhances cardiovascular endurance, reducing the risk of heart disease, stroke, and hypertension.

- Aerobic exercise increases heart rate and cardiac output, improving the efficiency of the cardiovascular system and enhancing overall heart health.

3. Calorie Burning and Weight Loss:

- Cardio exercise burns calories and promotes weight loss by increasing energy expenditure and creating a calorie deficit.

- Activities like running, cycling, swimming, and brisk walking can help burn calories, reduce body fat, and support weight management when combined with a balanced diet.

4. Endurance and Stamina:

- Regular cardio exercise improves aerobic capacity, endurance, and stamina, allowing individuals to sustain physical activity for longer durations without fatigue.

- Aerobic conditioning enhances the body's ability to utilize oxygen efficiently, delaying the onset of fatigue and improving performance in endurance activities.

5. Mental Health Benefits:

- Cardio exercise has numerous mental health benefits, including reducing stress, anxiety, and depression, and improving mood, cognitive function, and overall well-being.

- Aerobic activity stimulates the release of endorphins, neurotransmitters that promote feelings of happiness and relaxation, leading to improved mental health outcomes.

6. Metabolic Health:

- Cardiovascular exercise improves metabolic health by regulating blood sugar levels, enhancing insulin sensitivity, and reducing the risk of type 2 diabetes and metabolic syndrome.

- Regular aerobic activity can help control blood lipids, lower LDL cholesterol levels, and increase HDL cholesterol levels, improving lipid profiles and reducing cardiovascular risk factors.

7. Variety and Enjoyment:

- Cardio exercise offers a wide variety of activities to choose from, including indoor and outdoor options, group classes, team sports, and individual pursuits.

- Finding activities that you enjoy and that fit your fitness level and preferences can increase motivation, adherence, and long-term sustainability of your exercise routine.

Conclusion:

Strength training and cardio exercise offer distinct yet complementary benefits for overall health, fitness, and well-being. While strength training builds muscle strength, power, and endurance, cardio exercise improves cardiovascular fitness, endurance, and calorie burning. Incorporating both types of exercise into your routine can maximize the benefits and help you achieve a well-rounded fitness program. Whether you prefer lifting weights, running, cycling, swimming, or participating in group fitness classes, finding a balance between strength training and cardio can support your health and fitness goals and enhance your overall quality of life.

Stress Management

Stress management involves a variety of techniques and strategies aimed at reducing, coping with, and effectively managing stressors in order to promote overall well-being and resilience. In today's fast-paced world, where stressors are abundant and varied, learning how to manage stress effectively is essential for maintaining physical, mental, and emotional health. Here's an extensive and comprehensive overview of stress management techniques:

1. Identifying Stressors:

- The first step in stress management is identifying the sources of stress in your life. These stressors can be external (such as work deadlines, financial pressures, or relationship conflicts) or internal (such as negative self-talk, perfectionism, or unrealistic expectations).

- Keep a stress journal or diary to track your stressors and their impact on your thoughts, emotions, and behaviors. Recognizing patterns and triggers can help you develop effective coping strategies.

2. Developing Coping Skills:

- Coping skills are the tools and techniques you use to manage stress and navigate challenging situations effectively. There are various coping strategies to choose from, including:

- Problem-solving: Identify the specific problem or stressor and develop a plan of action to address it. Break the problem down into manageable steps and take proactive steps to find solutions.

- Emotional regulation: Learn to recognize and regulate your emotions in response to stress. Practice mindfulness, deep breathing, progressive muscle relaxation, or visualization techniques to calm the mind and body.

- Cognitive restructuring: Challenge negative or irrational thoughts and beliefs that contribute to stress and anxiety. Replace negative self-talk with more balanced and realistic thoughts.

- Seeking social support: Reach out to friends, family members, or support groups for emotional support and guidance. Talking to others who can empathize with your experiences can provide comfort and perspective.

- Time management: Prioritize tasks, set realistic goals, and establish boundaries to manage your time effectively. Break tasks down into smaller, more manageable steps and delegate responsibilities when possible.

- Healthy lifestyle habits: Maintain a balanced diet, engage in regular physical activity, prioritize sleep, and avoid excessive alcohol, caffeine, and substance use. Taking care of your physical health can improve your resilience to stress.

- Setting boundaries: Learn to say no to commitments or obligations that cause undue stress or overwhelm. Establish clear boundaries in your relationships and work-life balance to protect your time and energy.

3. Practicing Mindfulness and Relaxation Techniques:

- Mindfulness and relaxation techniques can help reduce stress by promoting a sense of calm, presence, and inner peace. Incorporate the following practices into your daily routine:

- Mindfulness meditation: Set aside time each day to practice mindfulness meditation, focusing your attention on the present moment without judgment. Pay attention to your breath, bodily sensations, and thoughts as they arise.

- Yoga and tai chi: Engage in gentle, flowing movements and breathwork to reduce stress and tension in the body. Yoga and tai chi promote relaxation, flexibility, and mind-body awareness.

- Progressive muscle relaxation: Tense and relax each muscle group in your body sequentially, starting from your toes and working your way up to your head. This technique can help release physical tension and promote relaxation.

- Deep breathing exercises: Practice diaphragmatic breathing or belly breathing to activate the body's relaxation response. Inhale deeply through your nose, filling your belly with air, and exhale slowly through your mouth, releasing tension and stress.

4. Engaging in Regular Physical Activity:

- Exercise is a powerful stress reliever that can improve mood, reduce anxiety, and promote relaxation. Aim for at least 150 minutes of moderate-intensity aerobic exercise or 75 minutes of vigorous-intensity aerobic exercise per week, along with two or more days of strength training exercises.

- Choose activities that you enjoy and that fit your fitness level and preferences, whether it's walking, jogging, cycling, swimming, dancing, or participating in group fitness classes. The key is to find activities that you find fun and engaging.

5. Practicing Self-Care and Healthy Lifestyle Habits:

- Self-care involves health professional.

- Therapy can provide a safe and supportive space to explore your thoughts, feelings, and coping strategies, and learn new skills for managing stress effectively.

- Consider cognitive-behavioral therapy (CBT), mindfulness-based stress reduction (MBSR), or other evidence-based approaches that address stress and anxiety.

7. Maintaining a Positive Outlook:

- Cultivate a positive mindset and optimistic outlook on life, even in the face of adversity. Focus on what you can control and influence, rather than dwelling on things beyond your control.

- Practice gratitude by reflecting on the things you're thankful for and expressing appreciation for the blessings in your life. Keeping a gratitude journal or practicing gratitude exercises can shift your perspective and promote feelings of positivity and resilience.

In conclusion, stress management involves a multifaceted approach that encompasses various techniques and strategies for reducing, coping with, and effectively managing stress. By identifying stressors, developing coping skills, practicing mindfulness and relaxation techniques, engaging in regular physical activity, prioritizing self-care and healthy lifestyle habits, seeking professional support when needed, and maintaining a positive outlook, you can cultivate resilience and enhance your overall well-being in the face of life's challenges. Experiment with different stress management techniques to find what works best for you, and prioritize self-care as an essential component of your daily routine.

Quality Sleep

Quality sleep is essential for overall health and well-being, playing a crucial role in physical, mental, and emotional functioning. Getting enough high-quality sleep is linked to numerous health benefits, including improved cognitive function, mood regulation, immune function, metabolism, and cardiovascular health. Here's an extensive and comprehensive overview of quality sleep:

1. Definition of Quality Sleep:
  - Quality sleep refers to sleep that is restorative, refreshing, and uninterrupted, allowing for the completion of essential sleep cycles and stages.

- It encompasses both the duration and the depth of sleep, as well as factors such as sleep efficiency, continuity, and subjective feelings of satisfaction upon waking.

2. Sleep Architecture and Stages:

- Sleep occurs in cycles that consist of multiple stages, each with unique characteristics and functions.

- The sleep cycle includes two main types of sleep: non-rapid eye movement (NREM) sleep and rapid eye movement (REM) sleep.

- NREM sleep is divided into three stages (N1, N2, and N3) characterized by progressively deeper levels of relaxation and restorative functions.

- REM sleep, also known as dream sleep, is associated with vivid dreams, cognitive processing, and memory consolidation.

3. Benefits of Quality Sleep:

- Cognitive function: Quality sleep enhances cognitive function, including memory consolidation, learning, problem-solving, decision-making, and creativity.

- Mood regulation: Adequate sleep promotes emotional well-being and resilience, reducing the risk of mood disorders such as depression and anxiety.

- Immune function: Quality sleep strengthens the immune system, helping to defend against infections and illnesses and support overall immune health.

- Metabolic health: Adequate sleep regulates appetite hormones, such as leptin and ghrelin, and supports metabolic function, reducing the risk of obesity, type 2 diabetes, and metabolic syndrome.

- Cardiovascular health: Quality sleep is associated with a lower risk of cardiovascular disease, hypertension, stroke, and other cardiovascular conditions.

- Physical recovery: Sleep is essential for physical recovery and repair, including muscle growth, tissue regeneration, hormone production, and cellular maintenance.

- Emotional regulation: Quality sleep helps regulate emotions, reduce stress, and promote resilience to emotional challenges and stressors.

4. Factors Affecting Sleep Quality:

- Several factors can influence the quality of sleep, including:

- Sleep environment: Comfortable bedding, a quiet, dark, and cool sleep environment, and minimal disruptions contribute to better sleep quality.

- Sleep hygiene: Establishing a regular sleep schedule, practicing relaxation techniques before bedtime, and avoiding stimulating activities, caffeine, and electronic devices close to bedtime promote better sleep hygiene.

- Stress and anxiety: Chronic stress, anxiety, and worry can disrupt sleep quality and lead to difficulty falling asleep, staying asleep, or experiencing restful sleep.

- Medical conditions: Certain medical conditions, such as sleep apnea, insomnia, restless legs syndrome, and chronic pain, can interfere with sleep quality and duration.

- Medications and substances: Some medications, caffeine, nicotine, alcohol, and recreational drugs can disrupt sleep patterns and impair sleep quality.

- Mental health: Mental health disorders, such as depression, anxiety, and post-traumatic stress disorder (PTSD), can affect sleep quality and contribute to sleep disturbances.

5. Strategies for Improving Sleep Quality:

- Establish a consistent sleep schedule: Go to bed and wake up at the same time every day, even on weekends, to regulate your body's internal clock and promote better sleep quality.

- Create a relaxing bedtime routine: Develop a calming pre-sleep routine that signals to your body that it's time to wind down. This may include activities such as reading, taking a warm bath, practicing relaxation techniques, or listening to soothing music.

- Optimize your sleep environment: Make your bedroom conducive to sleep by creating a dark, quiet, and comfortable sleep environment. Invest in a supportive mattress and pillows, use blackout curtains or eye masks to block out light, and use white noise machines or earplugs to minimize noise disruptions.

- Practice good sleep hygiene: Avoid stimulants like caffeine and nicotine close to bedtime, limit screen time and exposure to electronic devices, and create a relaxing bedtime ritual to prepare your body and mind for sleep.

- Manage stress and anxiety: Practice stress-reduction techniques such as mindfulness meditation, deep breathing exercises, progressive muscle relaxation, or journaling to calm the mind and promote relaxation before bedtime.

- Exercise regularly: Engage in regular physical activity, but avoid vigorous exercise close to bedtime, as it can be stimulating and interfere with sleep. Aim for moderate-intensity exercise earlier in the day to promote better sleep quality.

- Monitor your sleep patterns: Keep a sleep diary or use sleep tracking apps or devices to monitor your sleep patterns and identify factors that may be affecting your sleep quality. This can help you identify patterns, track improvements, and make adjustments to your sleep habits as needed.

- Seek professional help if needed: If you continue to experience persistent sleep problems despite implementing healthy sleep habits, consider seeking guidance from a healthcare professional or sleep specialist. They can help diagnose and treat underlying sleep disorders or medical conditions that may be contributing to poor sleep quality.

In conclusion, quality sleep is essential for overall health, well-being, and functioning. By prioritizing sleep hygiene, creating a relaxing sleep environment, managing stress and anxiety, and adopting healthy sleep habits, you can improve the quality and duration of your sleep and reap the numerous benefits of restorative rest. Remember that quality sleep is a fundamental pillar of health and should be treated as a priority in your daily routine.

Chapter 8:

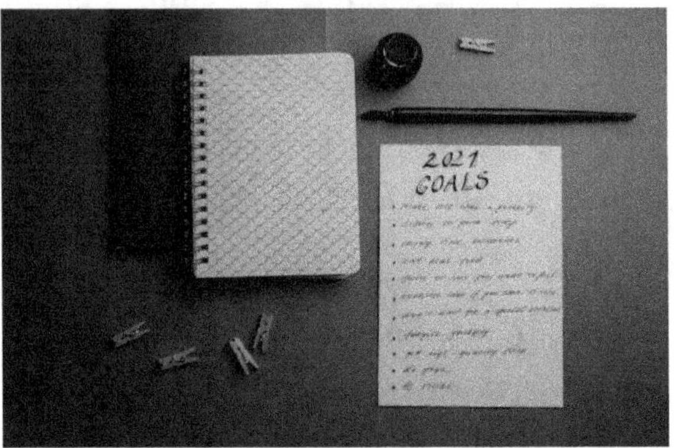

Tracking Progress and Adjusting Your Approach

Tracking progress and adjusting your approach are essential components of any goal-oriented endeavor, whether it's improving fitness, managing weight, developing a new skill, or achieving personal or professional milestones. By monitoring your progress, identifying areas for improvement, and making adjustments as needed, you can optimize your efforts, stay motivated, and ultimately increase your chances of success. Here's an extensive and comprehensive overview of tracking progress and adjusting your approach:

1. Setting Clear Goals:

- The first step in tracking progress is establishing clear, specific, and measurable goals that align with your values, priorities, and aspirations.

- Define what success looks like for you, whether it's running a certain distance, losing a specific amount of weight, mastering a skill, or achieving a professional milestone.

- Break larger goals down into smaller, more manageable milestones or action steps that you can track and measure over time.

2. Choosing Relevant Metrics:

- Select metrics or indicators that are relevant to your goals and reflect your progress accurately. This may include quantitative measures (e.g., distance, time, weight, repetitions) and qualitative measures (e.g., skill proficiency, subjective ratings, self-assessments).

- Consider using a combination of objective data (e.g., measurements, performance metrics) and subjective feedback (e.g., self-assessments, journal entries) to gain a comprehensive understanding of your progress.

3. Establishing Baselines:

- Before you begin tracking progress, establish baseline measurements or assessments to benchmark your starting point.

- Take initial measurements, conduct fitness assessments, or perform skill evaluations to establish a baseline against which you can compare future progress.

- Baseline data provides context for your progress and allows you to track improvements over time.

4. Implementing Tracking Systems:

- Choose tracking methods and systems that are convenient, accessible, and compatible with your goals and preferences.

- Utilize various tools and technologies to track progress, including fitness apps, wearable devices, spreadsheets, journals, or online platforms.

- Regularly input data, record observations, or update your tracking system to maintain accurate and up-to-date records of your progress.

5. Monitoring Progress Regularly:

- Consistently monitor your progress at regular intervals to track changes over time and identify trends, patterns, or areas for improvement.

- Set aside dedicated time to review your progress, analyze data, and reflect on your achievements and challenges.

- Adjust your tracking frequency based on the nature of your goals and the rate of progress, ranging from daily or weekly check-ins to monthly or quarterly evaluations.

6.Analyzing Results and Identifying Trends:

- Analyze your progress data to identify trends, patterns, strengths, and areas for improvement.

- Look for consistent improvements, plateaus, or setbacks in your metrics and assess factors that may have contributed to changes in performance.

- Consider qualitative feedback, subjective experiences, and external factors that may influence your progress, such as lifestyle habits, environmental conditions, or external stressors.

7. Celebrating Achievements and Milestones:

- Acknowledge and celebrate your achievements, milestones, and progress along the way to stay motivated and reinforce positive behaviors.

- Recognize your hard work, dedication, and perseverance, regardless of the size or significance of the accomplishment.

- Celebrate progress milestones with rewards, incentives, or meaningful experiences that reinforce your commitment and progress.

8. Making Adjustments and Course Corrections:

- Based on your progress analysis, identify areas where adjustments or course corrections may be necessary to optimize your approach.

- Modify your goals, strategies, or action plans as needed to address challenges, overcome obstacles, or capitalize on opportunities for improvement.

- Be flexible and open-minded in adapting your approach, and be willing to experiment with new techniques, strategies, or interventions to achieve your goals.

9. Seeking Feedback and Support:

- Solicit feedback from trusted sources, mentors, coaches, or peers to gain additional perspectives on your progress and performance.

- Consult with experts, professionals, or individuals with relevant experience to seek guidance, advice, or recommendations for optimizing your approach.

- Surround yourself with a supportive network of friends, family members, or colleagues who can provide encouragement, accountability, and constructive feedback.

10. Maintaining Motivation and Persistence:

- Stay motivated and resilient in the face of setbacks, challenges, or obstacles by focusing on your long-term goals and aspirations.

- Use setbacks as opportunities for learning and growth, rather than reasons for discouragement or defeat.

- Cultivate a growth mindset, positive attitude, and determination to persevere in the pursuit of your goals, regardless of obstacles or setbacks.

11. Iterating and Refining Your Approach:

- Continuously iterate and refine your approach based on ongoing feedback, experience, and insights gained from tracking progress.

- Embrace a process of continuous improvement, learning, and adaptation to optimize your strategies and maximize your chances of success.

- Remain flexible and responsive to changing circumstances, evolving priorities, and new information that may impact your goals and approach.

In conclusion, tracking progress and adjusting your approach are essential components of achieving success and reaching your goals. By setting clear goals, choosing relevant metrics, establishing baselines, implementing tracking systems, monitoring progress regularly, analyzing results, celebrating achievements, making adjustments, seeking feedback and support, maintaining motivation and persistence, and iterating and refining your approach, you can optimize your efforts and increase your likelihood of success. Remember that progress is not always linear, and setbacks are a natural part of the journey. Stay committed, resilient, and adaptable, and keep moving forward toward your goals with determination and perseverance.

Setting Realistic Goals

Setting realistic goals is a foundational step in personal and professional development. Realistic goals are those that are achievable, meaningful, and aligned with your capabilities, resources, and circumstances. Whether you're aiming to improve your health, advance your career, learn a new skill, or pursue personal growth, setting realistic goals increases your likelihood of success and empowers you to make tangible progress toward your aspirations. Here's an extensive and comprehensive guide on setting realistic goals:

Understanding the Importance of Realistic Goals:

1. Clarity and Direction: Realistic goals provide clarity and direction by outlining specific objectives or outcomes that you want to achieve.

2. Motivation and Focus: Realistic goals serve as sources of motivation and focus, guiding your efforts and actions toward meaningful results.

3. Accountability and Progress Tracking: Realistic goals hold you accountable for your actions and enable you to track your progress effectively, allowing you to adjust your approach as needed.

4. Confidence Building: Achieving realistic goals boosts your confidence and self-esteem, reinforcing your belief in your abilities and increasing your motivation to pursue future goals.

Characteristics of Realistic Goals:

1. Specificity: Realistic goals are clear and specific, clearly defining what you want to accomplish and how you plan to achieve it.

2. Achievability: Realistic goals are attainable within a reasonable timeframe and with the available resources, skills, and support systems.

3. Relevance: Realistic goals are relevant to your values, priorities, and long-term objectives, aligning with your personal or professional aspirations.

4. Time-Bound: Realistic goals have a defined timeframe or deadline for completion, providing a sense of urgency and focus.

Factors to Consider When Setting Realistic Goals:

1. Personal Capabilities: Consider your strengths, weaknesses, skills, and experience when setting goals, ensuring they are within your capabilities.

2. Available Resources: Assess the resources, support systems, and tools at your disposal, ensuring your goals are feasible within your constraints.

3. Current Circumstances: Take into account your current circumstances, including external factors and commitments, when setting goals.

4. Past Experiences: Reflect on past successes, failures, and lessons learned to set realistic expectations and inform your goal-setting process.

Strategies for Setting Realistic Goals:

1. Break Goals Down: Divide larger goals into smaller, more manageable tasks or milestones to make them easier to achieve and track progress effectively.

2. SMART Criteria: Apply the SMART criteria (Specific, Measurable, Achievable, Relevant, Time-bound) to ensure your goals are well-defined and achievable.

3. Prioritize Goals: Identify and prioritize goals based on their importance, urgency, and potential impact on your life or work.

4. Review and Revise Regularly: Review your goals regularly to assess progress, make adjustments, and ensure alignment with changing circumstances or priorities.

Examples of Realistic Goals:

1. Health and Fitness: Aim to exercise for 30 minutes, three times per week, gradually increasing intensity and duration over time.

2. Career Advancement: Set a goal to acquire a new skill or certification within a specific timeframe to enhance your qualifications and career prospects.

3. Financial Savings: Set a goal to save a certain amount of money each month toward a

specific financial goal, such as building an emergency fund or paying off debt.

4. Personal Development: Commit to reading one book per month in a subject area that interests you, or learn a new hobby or skill that you've always wanted to pursue.

5. Relationship Improvement: Schedule regular quality time with your partner or family members to strengthen your relationships and foster connection.

Tips for Achieving Realistic Goals:

1. Break Goals Down: Divide larger goals into smaller, more manageable tasks or action steps to make progress more achievable and sustainable.

2. Stay Focused and Disciplined: Maintain focus on your goals by prioritizing tasks,

managing distractions, and staying disciplined in your efforts.

3. Seek Support and Accountability: Share your goals with trusted friends, family members, or mentors who can provide encouragement, guidance, and accountability.

4. Celebrate Progress: Acknowledge and celebrate your progress, no matter how small, to stay motivated and reinforce positive behaviors.

5. Adjust Your Approach: Be flexible and willing to adjust your approach based on feedback, changing circumstances, or new information.

Conclusion:

Setting realistic goals is essential for achieving success and personal growth. By following the strategies outlined above and avoiding common mistakes, you can set yourself up for success and make steady progress toward your aspirations. Remember that goal-setting is a dynamic process, and it's okay to adjust your goals as needed along the way. Stay focused, stay positive, and stay committed to your journey of growth and achievement.

Monitoring Changes in Weight and Body Composition

Monitoring changes in weight and body composition is essential for individuals looking to manage their health, fitness, or weight loss goals effectively. By regularly tracking changes in weight, body fat percentage, muscle mass, and other relevant metrics, you can assess your progress, adjust your approach as needed, and stay motivated on your journey toward better health and well-being. Here's an extensive and comprehensive guide on monitoring changes in weight and body composition:

Importance of Monitoring Changes:

1. Assessment of Progress: Regular monitoring allows you to assess your progress toward your health or fitness goals, helping you determine whether your current approach is working effectively.

2. Identification of Trends: Tracking changes over time helps you identify trends and patterns in your weight and body composition, allowing you to make informed decisions about your diet, exercise, and lifestyle habits.

3. Motivation and Accountability: Monitoring progress provides motivation and accountability, as seeing positive changes can inspire you to stay committed to your goals and make necessary adjustments along the way.

4. Early Detection of Issues: Monitoring allows you to detect any deviations from your desired trajectory early on, enabling you to address potential issues before they become more significant challenges.

Metrics for Monitoring Changes:

1. Weight: Tracking changes in body weight is a straightforward way to monitor progress. However, it's essential to recognize that fluctuations in weight can occur due to factors such as hydration levels, food intake, and time of day.

2. Body Fat Percentage: Measuring body fat percentage provides a more accurate assessment of changes in body composition than weight alone. Methods for measuring body fat percentage include bioelectrical impedance analysis (BIA), skinfold calipers, DEXA scans, and underwater weighing.

3. Muscle Mass: Monitoring changes in muscle mass is crucial for individuals focusing on strength training or body recomposition goals. While methods for measuring muscle mass vary, techniques such as BIA and DEXA scans can provide valuable insights.

4. Waist Circumference: Waist circumference is an indicator of abdominal fat and visceral adiposity, both of which are associated with an increased risk of metabolic disorders such as type 2 diabetes and cardiovascular disease.

5. Other Body Measurements: Additional measurements, such as hip circumference, thigh circumference, and body circumferences, can provide insights into changes in body shape and distribution of fat and muscle mass.

Frequency of Monitoring:

1. Regular Schedule: Establish a regular schedule for monitoring changes in weight and body composition. Depending on your goals and preferences, this may range from weekly to monthly assessments.

2. Consistency: To ensure accurate and reliable measurements, maintain consistency in the timing and conditions of your assessments. For example, weigh yourself at the same time of day, under similar conditions (e.g., after waking up and using the bathroom), and using the same scale.

Methods for Monitoring Changes:

1. Body Weight Scales: Digital scales are readily available and offer a convenient way to monitor changes in weight at home. Look for scales that also provide body composition metrics, such as body fat percentage and muscle mass.

2. Body Composition Analyzers: Bioelectrical impedance analysis (BIA) devices use electrical signals to estimate body composition. These devices are available in various forms, including handheld devices, scales with built-in BIA technology, and professional-grade equipment.

3. Skinfold Calipers: Skinfold calipers measure the thickness of skinfolds at specific sites on the body to estimate body fat percentage. While less accurate than some other methods,

skinfold calipers can still provide useful information when used correctly.

4. DEXA Scans: Dual-energy X-ray absorptiometry (DEXA) scans are considered the gold standard for assessing body composition. These scans provide detailed information about bone density, fat mass, and lean mass distribution.

Interpreting Changes:

1. Long-Term Trends: Focus on long-term trends rather than day-to-day fluctuations. Small changes in weight or body composition over time are often more meaningful than short-term fluctuations.

2. Set Realistic Expectations: Recognize that progress may occur gradually and may not always be linear. Set realistic expectations and celebrate small victories along the way.

3. Consider Multiple Metrics: Instead of relying solely on weight as a measure of progress, consider multiple metrics, such as body fat percentage, muscle mass, and waist circumference, to get a more comprehensive picture of changes in body composition.

4. Seek Professional Guidance: If you're unsure how to interpret changes in weight or body composition, or if you have specific health or fitness goals, consider seeking guidance from a healthcare professional, nutritionist, or fitness trainer.

Adjusting Your Approach:

1. Evaluate Your Strategy: Periodically review your diet, exercise routine, and lifestyle habits to assess their effectiveness in achieving your goals.

2. Make Informed Changes: Use the information gathered from monitoring changes in weight and body composition to make informed decisions about adjustments to your approach.

3. Seek Support and Accountability: Share your progress and goals with a supportive community, such as friends, family, or online forums, to gain encouragement, accountability, and guidance.

4. Be Patient and Persistent: Remember that achieving meaningful changes in weight and body composition takes time, patience, and consistent effort. Stay committed to your goals and trust in the process.

Conclusion:

Monitoring changes in weight and body composition is an essential aspect of health, fitness, and weight management. By regularly assessing your progress, using reliable metrics, and interpreting changes accurately, you can make informed decisions about your diet, exercise, and lifestyle habits. Whether your goal is to lose weight, build muscle, or improve overall health, tracking changes in weight and body composition empowers you to stay motivated, adjust your approach as needed, and make meaningful progress toward your goals. Remember to focus on long-term trends, set realistic expectations, and celebrate your achievements along the way. With dedication, consistency, and a proactive approach to monitoring changes, you can optimize your health and well-being over time.

Making Adjustments for Long-Term Success

Making adjustments for long-term success is crucial for individuals striving to achieve their goals and maintain progress over time. Whether you're pursuing health and fitness objectives, career aspirations, personal development goals, or any other endeavor, adapting your approach as circumstances change and challenges arise is essential for sustained success. Here's an extensive and comprehensive guide on making adjustments for long-term success:

Understanding the Need for Adjustments:

1. Dynamic Nature of Goals: Recognize that goals and circumstances are dynamic, evolving over time due to various factors such as

personal growth, changing priorities, and external influences.

2. Overcoming Challenges: Making adjustments allows you to overcome obstacles, setbacks, and unexpected challenges that may arise on your journey toward your goals.

3. Optimizing Strategies: Adapting your approach enables you to optimize your strategies, capitalize on opportunities, and refine your methods for greater effectiveness.

4. Maintaining Motivation: By making adjustments when necessary, you can maintain motivation, prevent stagnation, and sustain progress toward your long-term objectives.

Signs That Adjustments Are Needed:

1. Plateauing Progress: If you've reached a plateau or are experiencing stagnant progress, it may be time to reassess your approach and make necessary changes.

2. Lack of Satisfaction: Feeling dissatisfied or unfulfilled despite making efforts toward your goals can indicate the need for adjustments to align your actions with your values and aspirations.

3. Changes in Circumstances: Significant life changes, such as career shifts, personal transitions, or health-related issues, may necessitate adjustments to your goals and strategies.

4. Feedback and Reflection: Feedback from others, self-reflection, and periodic assessments of your progress can provide insights into areas where adjustments may be beneficial.

Strategies for Making Adjustments:

1. Evaluate Your Current Approach: Reflect on your goals, strategies, and progress to identify areas where adjustments may be needed. Consider what's working well and what could be improved.

2. Set Clear Objectives: Define specific objectives for the adjustments you plan to make, ensuring they are aligned with your long-term goals and priorities.

3. Be Flexible and Open-Minded: Embrace flexibility and openness to change, recognizing that adjustments are a natural part of the journey toward success.

4. Gather Information: Gather information, seek advice from experts or mentors, and explore

different perspectives to inform your decision-making process.

5. Prioritize Changes: Prioritize adjustments based on their potential impact on your goals and the feasibility of implementation within your current circumstances.

6. Implement Changes Gradually: Introduce changes gradually to allow for adaptation and minimize disruption to your routine. Monitor the effects of each adjustment and make further modifications as needed.

Examples of Adjustments:

1. Health and Fitness Goals:
   - Adjusting your workout routine to include different exercises or increase intensity.
   - Modifying your dietary habits to address changing nutritional needs or preferences.

2. Career Goals:

- Pursuing additional education or training to enhance your skills and qualifications.

- Networking and seeking new opportunities for career advancement or professional development.

3. Personal Development Goals:

- Setting new objectives or milestones to challenge yourself and foster growth.

- Seeking feedback from peers or mentors to identify areas for improvement.

4. Relationship Goals:

- Communicating openly with your partner or loved ones to address conflicts or strengthen connections.

- Investing time and effort into nurturing relationships and building a supportive social network.

Tips for Long-Term Success:

1. Stay Committed: Maintain commitment and perseverance, even when faced with setbacks or challenges along the way.

2. Stay Flexible: Embrace flexibility and adaptability, being willing to adjust your approach as needed to overcome obstacles and achieve your goals.

3. Seek Support: Seek support from friends, family, mentors, or professionals who can provide guidance, encouragement, and accountability.

4. Celebrate Progress: Acknowledge and celebrate your achievements, no matter how small, to stay motivated and reinforce positive behaviors.

5. Stay Focused on Your Why: Keep your overarching goals and motivations in mind,

reminding yourself why you embarked on this journey in the first place.

Conclusion:

Making adjustments for long-term success is essential for achieving your goals and sustaining progress over time. By recognizing the need for adjustments, evaluating your current approach, and implementing changes strategically, you can overcome challenges, optimize your strategies, and maintain momentum toward your objectives. Embrace flexibility, stay committed to your goals, and seek support when needed to navigate obstacles and achieve lasting success in your endeavors. With a proactive and adaptive mindset, you can overcome obstacles, adapt to changing circumstances, and ultimately achieve your long-term aspirations.

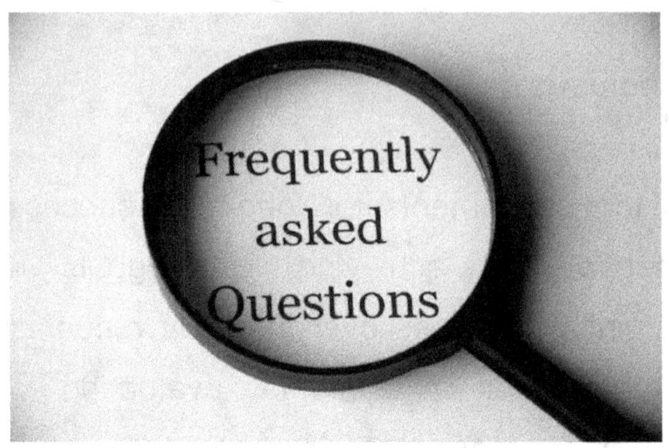

Frequently Asked Questions about Fat-Burning Foods and Metabolism

Certainly! Here's an extensive and comprehensive list of frequently asked questions about fat-burning foods and metabolism:

1. What are fat-burning foods?

Fat-burning foods are foods that have properties believed to enhance metabolism and promote fat loss. These foods are often rich in nutrients, fiber, and/or compounds that may increase energy expenditure or promote satiety.

2. How do fat-burning foods work?

Fat-burning foods can work through various mechanisms, such as boosting metabolism, increasing satiety, stabilizing blood sugar levels, and promoting fat oxidation. Some foods may contain compounds that enhance thermogenesis or increase the body's calorie-burning process.

3. Do fat-burning foods really help with weight loss?

While fat-burning foods can contribute to weight loss when included as part of a balanced diet and healthy lifestyle, they are not a magic solution for shedding excess pounds. Weight loss ultimately depends on creating a calorie deficit, which can be achieved through a combination of dietary changes, physical activity, and lifestyle modifications.

4. What are some examples of fat-burning foods?

Examples of fat-burning foods include lean proteins (such as chicken breast, fish, and tofu), fruits and vegetables (particularly those high in fiber and water content), whole grains, nuts and seeds, green tea, and spicy foods containing capsaicin.

5. Are there specific foods that target belly fat?

While spot reduction of fat is not possible, certain foods and dietary patterns may help reduce overall body fat, including abdominal fat. Foods rich in soluble fiber, healthy fats, and protein can help promote feelings of fullness and support weight loss, which may help reduce belly fat over time.

6. Can certain foods speed up metabolism?

Some foods, such as those high in protein, fiber, and certain spices, may temporarily increase metabolism through the thermic effect of food (TEF) or by stimulating metabolic processes. However, the overall impact of dietary factors on metabolism is relatively small compared to factors such as age, gender, genetics, and physical activity level.

7. Is it necessary to eat small, frequent meals to boost metabolism?

There is no one-size-fits-all approach to meal frequency for boosting metabolism. Some individuals may prefer eating smaller, more frequent meals, while others may thrive on larger, less frequent meals. The most important factor is to maintain a balanced diet that provides adequate nutrients and supports overall health and well-being.

8. How does metabolism change with age?

Metabolism tends to decrease with age, primarily due to a decline in muscle mass, changes in hormone levels, and decreased physical activity. However, adopting healthy lifestyle habits, such as regular exercise and a balanced diet, can help mitigate age-related declines in metabolism and maintain overall health.

9. Are there any side effects of consuming fat-burning foods?

While fat-burning foods are generally safe and nutritious when consumed as part of a balanced diet, some individuals may experience digestive discomfort or allergic reactions to certain foods. Additionally, consuming excessive amounts of spicy foods or stimulants such as caffeine may cause gastrointestinal upset or other adverse effects in sensitive individuals.

10. Can supplements help boost metabolism?

While certain supplements claim to enhance metabolism or promote fat loss, their effectiveness and safety can vary widely. It's essential to approach supplements with caution and consult with a healthcare professional before taking them, as some may have unwanted side effects or interact with medications.

11. How important is physical activity for boosting metabolism?

Physical activity plays a crucial role in boosting metabolism by increasing energy expenditure, preserving lean muscle mass, and promoting overall health and well-being. Incorporating regular exercise, including both cardiovascular and strength training activities, is essential for maintaining a healthy metabolism and supporting weight management efforts.

12. Are there specific foods to avoid for weight loss?

While no single food should be entirely off-limits, it's generally advisable to limit or avoid highly processed foods, sugary snacks and beverages, fried foods, and foods high in saturated and trans fats. Instead, focus on whole, nutrient-dense foods that support overall health and promote satiety.

Conclusion:

Understanding the role of fat-burning foods and metabolism is essential for making informed dietary choices and supporting weight management goals. While fat-burning foods can be beneficial as part of a balanced diet and healthy lifestyle, they are just one piece of the puzzle when it comes to achieving and maintaining a healthy weight. By focusing on overall dietary patterns, regular physical activity, and sustainable lifestyle habits, individuals can optimize their metabolism and support long-term health and well-being.

Can certain foods really boost metabolism?

The concept of certain foods boosting metabolism is a topic of interest for many individuals seeking to optimize their health, support weight management efforts, and enhance energy expenditure. While some foods may have modest effects on metabolism, it's essential to understand the science behind this phenomenon and manage expectations regarding their impact. Here's an extensive and comprehensive exploration of whether certain foods can truly boost metabolism:

Understanding Metabolism:

1. Basal Metabolic Rate (BMR): Metabolism refers to the chemical processes that occur within the body to maintain life. Basal metabolic rate (BMR) represents the energy expended at rest to maintain essential bodily functions, such as breathing, circulation, and cell repair.

2. Thermic Effect of Food (TEF): The thermic effect of food (TEF) refers to the energy expenditure associated with digesting, absorbing, and metabolizing nutrients from food. Different macronutrients have varying TEF percentages, with protein typically requiring more energy to metabolize than carbohydrates or fats.

3. Physical Activity and Exercise: Physical activity, including exercise, contributes to total energy expenditure by burning calories above and beyond BMR and TEF. Both aerobic

(cardio) and anaerobic (strength training) exercise can impact metabolism by increasing muscle mass, which in turn raises BMR.

The Role of Certain Foods:

1. Protein-Rich Foods: Protein is known to have a higher thermic effect compared to carbohydrates and fats, meaning it requires more energy to digest and metabolize. Including protein-rich foods such as lean meats, fish, eggs, dairy products, legumes, and tofu in your diet can potentially increase energy expenditure and support weight management efforts.

2. Foods High in Fiber: Fiber-rich foods, such as fruits, vegetables, whole grains, legumes, and nuts, are often associated with increased satiety and improved digestive health. While fiber itself does not significantly impact metabolism directly, its role in promoting

feelings of fullness may indirectly support weight management by reducing calorie intake.

3. Spicy Foods: Some research suggests that compounds found in spicy foods, such as capsaicin in chili peppers, may temporarily increase metabolism and promote fat oxidation. However, the effects are typically modest and may vary among individuals.

4. Green Tea: Green tea contains catechins and caffeine, compounds that have been studied for their potential thermogenic and fat-burning effects. While research on the metabolic effects of green tea is mixed, some studies suggest that consuming green tea may modestly increase calorie expenditure and fat oxidation.

Factors to Consider:

1. Individual Variability: Metabolic responses to foods can vary widely among individuals due to factors such as genetics, age, gender, body composition, and overall health status. What works for one person may not have the same effect on another.

2. Overall Dietary Pattern: Rather than focusing solely on individual foods, it's essential to consider the overall dietary pattern and lifestyle habits. A balanced diet that includes a variety of nutrient-dense foods, along with regular physical activity, is key to supporting metabolism and overall health.

3. Caloric Balance: Ultimately, weight management and metabolic health depend on achieving a balance between caloric intake and expenditure. While certain foods may have metabolic benefits, they should be incorporated as part of a well-rounded diet that aligns with overall energy needs and goals.

4. Sustainability: Sustainable dietary habits that can be maintained long-term are more important than short-term fixes. Instead of relying on specific "metabolism-boosting" foods, focus on building a healthy, balanced eating pattern that you can enjoy and sustain over time.

Conclusion:

While certain foods may have the potential to modestly impact metabolism through mechanisms such as increasing thermogenesis or promoting satiety, their effects should be considered within the broader context of overall dietary patterns and lifestyle habits. Incorporating protein-rich foods, fiber-rich foods, spicy foods, and green tea into your diet can be part of a healthy eating plan that supports metabolic health and weight management. However, sustainable lifestyle changes, including regular physical activity and mindful eating practices, are essential for long-term success. Instead of searching for quick fixes or magic solutions, focus on nurturing a balanced approach to nutrition and wellness that promotes overall health and well-being.

How long does it take to see results?

The time it takes to see results from efforts such as diet changes, exercise routines, or lifestyle modifications can vary widely depending on various factors, including individual circumstances, goals, and the specific interventions implemented. While some individuals may notice changes relatively quickly, others may experience a more gradual progression over time. Here's an extensive and comprehensive exploration of the factors influencing the timeline for seeing results:

Factors Influencing Time to See Results:

1. Individual Characteristics: Each person's body is unique, with different genetic factors, metabolic rates, body compositions, and health statuses. These individual differences can influence how quickly or slowly changes occur in response to diet and exercise interventions.

2. Starting Point: The starting point plays a significant role in determining the timeline for seeing results. Individuals who are starting from a healthier baseline may notice changes more quickly than those who have significant weight to lose or underlying health conditions to address.

3. Specific Goals: The nature of the goals can also affect the timeline for seeing results. For example, goals related to weight loss, muscle gain, cardiovascular fitness, flexibility, or

endurance may each have different timelines for noticeable improvements.

4. Consistency and Compliance: Consistency and adherence to the chosen interventions are crucial for achieving results. Consistently following a well-designed diet plan, sticking to an exercise routine, and making sustainable lifestyle changes are essential for seeing progress over time.

5. Intensity and Duration: The intensity and duration of the interventions can impact how quickly results are achieved. More intense or longer-duration workouts, stricter dietary changes, or more significant lifestyle modifications may yield faster results but may also be more challenging to sustain.

6. Health Conditions: Underlying health conditions, such as metabolic disorders, hormonal imbalances, or chronic diseases, can

affect the body's response to interventions and may influence the timeline for seeing results.

Typical Timelines for Seeing Results:

1. Weight Loss: While weight loss can vary widely depending on individual factors, a safe and sustainable rate of weight loss is typically considered to be 1-2 pounds per week. Therefore, noticeable changes in weight may be observed within a few weeks to a few months, depending on the amount of weight to lose and the adherence to dietary and exercise recommendations.

2. Muscle Gain: Building muscle mass typically takes longer than losing weight. Visible changes in muscle tone and definition may be observed within a few months of consistent strength training exercises, but significant muscle growth may take several months to years to achieve, especially for beginners.

3. Improved Fitness: Cardiovascular fitness, strength, endurance, and flexibility can all improve with regular exercise over time. Depending on the starting fitness level and the intensity of the exercise program, noticeable improvements in fitness may be observed within a few weeks to a few months.

4. Health Markers: Changes in health markers such as blood pressure, cholesterol levels, blood sugar levels, and overall well-being may occur relatively quickly with improvements in diet and exercise habits. However, it may take several months to see significant changes in these markers, especially for individuals with chronic health conditions.

Tips for Maximizing Results:

1. Set Realistic Expectations: Understand that meaningful changes take time and patience.

Focus on making sustainable lifestyle changes rather than expecting immediate results.

2. Track Progress: Keep track of your progress through methods such as taking measurements, recording workouts, or keeping a food diary. Monitoring changes over time can help you stay motivated and identify areas for improvement.

3. Stay Consistent: Consistency is key for seeing results. Stick to your chosen interventions even when progress feels slow, and trust the process.

4. Listen to Your Body: Pay attention to how your body responds to diet and exercise changes. Rest when needed, adjust your approach as necessary, and seek guidance from healthcare professionals or fitness experts if you encounter challenges.

5. Celebrate Small Wins: Acknowledge and celebrate small victories along the way, whether it's reaching a fitness milestone, fitting into a smaller clothing size, or feeling more energized and confident.

Conclusion:

The timeline for seeing results from diet, exercise, and lifestyle changes varies from person to person and depends on various factors such as individual characteristics, goals, consistency, and starting point. While some changes may be noticeable relatively quickly, significant and sustainable results often take time, patience, and dedication. By setting realistic expectations, staying consistent, and focusing on long-term progress rather than short-term outcomes, individuals can maximize their chances of achieving their desired goals and maintaining their health and well-being over time.

Are there any side effects to consider?

When implementing diet changes, exercise routines, or lifestyle modifications, it's essential to be aware of potential side effects that may arise. While many interventions aimed at improving health and well-being can have positive effects, it's also possible to experience adverse reactions or unintended consequences. Here's an extensive and comprehensive exploration of the potential side effects to consider:

Dietary Changes:

1. Caloric Restriction: If implementing a calorie-restricted diet for weight loss, some individuals may experience side effects such as hunger,

irritability, fatigue, or dizziness, especially during the initial phase of adjustment.

2. Nutrient Deficiencies: Restrictive diets or elimination diets may increase the risk of nutrient deficiencies, particularly if certain food groups are excluded. Common deficiencies may include iron, calcium, vitamin D, vitamin B12, and omega-3 fatty acids.

3. Digestive Discomfort: Introducing new foods or dietary fibers may lead to digestive discomfort, such as bloating, gas, or diarrhea, as the gut microbiota adjusts to the changes in dietary composition.

4. Food Sensitivities or Allergies: Some individuals may have sensitivities or allergies to specific foods, leading to adverse reactions such as skin rashes, digestive issues, or respiratory symptoms.

Exercise Routines:

1. Muscle Soreness: Introducing a new exercise routine or increasing the intensity of workouts may result in delayed-onset muscle soreness (DOMS), characterized by stiffness, tenderness, and discomfort in the muscles.

2. Overuse Injuries: Overexertion or repetitive movements without adequate rest and recovery may increase the risk of overuse injuries, such as tendinitis, stress fractures, or muscle strains.

3. Fatigue and Burnout: Pushing too hard without allowing sufficient rest and recovery may lead to fatigue, burnout, or even overtraining syndrome, characterized by persistent fatigue, decreased performance, and mood disturbances.

4. Joint Pain: High-impact exercises or improper form during strength training may exacerbate joint pain or lead to injuries, particularly in individuals with pre-existing joint conditions or musculoskeletal issues.

Lifestyle Modifications:

1. Sleep Disturbances: Changes in sleep habits, such as adopting a new sleep schedule or reducing screen time before bed, may initially disrupt sleep patterns and result in insomnia or sleep disturbances.

2. Stress and Anxiety: Making significant lifestyle changes, such as starting a new job, moving to a new location, or altering daily routines, can be stressful and may contribute to feelings of anxiety or overwhelm.

3. Social Impact: Altering dietary habits or exercise routines may affect social interactions,

particularly in settings where food or physical activity plays a central role, leading to feelings of isolation or social discomfort.

4.Emotional Well-being: Changes in diet, exercise, or lifestyle habits may impact emotional well-being and mood, especially if individuals struggle with body image issues, disordered eating patterns, or mental health conditions.

Managing Side Effects:

1. **Gradual Progression**: Introduce changes gradually to allow the body to adapt and minimize the risk of adverse reactions. Slowly increase exercise intensity, gradually modify dietary habits, and prioritize rest and recovery.

2. Listen to Your Body: Pay attention to signs and symptoms that your body may be experiencing adverse effects, such as fatigue,

pain, or digestive discomfort. Adjust your approach accordingly and seek guidance from healthcare professionals if needed.

3. Balance and Moderation: Strive for balance and moderation in all aspects of health and wellness. Avoid extremes in diet or exercise and prioritize sustainable lifestyle habits that support overall well-being.

4. Seek Support: Don't hesitate to seek support from healthcare professionals, nutritionists, fitness trainers, or mental health professionals if you encounter challenges or need assistance in managing side effects.

Conclusion:

While diet changes, exercise routines, and lifestyle modifications can have numerous benefits for health and well-being, it's essential to be mindful of potential side effects that may arise. By understanding the potential risks, listening to your body, and implementing changes gradually and mindfully, you can minimize adverse reactions and maximize the positive effects of your health and wellness journey. Remember that every individual is unique, so what works well for one person may not be suitable for another. Prioritize your health and well-being, and seek support as needed to navigate any challenges along the way.

Can metabolism be permanently boosted?

The concept of "boosting" metabolism often conjures up images of quick fixes or magic solutions to achieve rapid weight loss or increased energy expenditure. While certain factors can temporarily influence metabolism, such as dietary changes, exercise, and lifestyle modifications, the idea of permanently boosting metabolism is more nuanced. Here's an extensive and comprehensive exploration of whether metabolism can be permanently boosted:

Understanding Metabolism:

1. Basal Metabolic Rate (BMR): Metabolism refers to the complex series of biochemical processes that occur within the body to sustain life. Basal metabolic rate (BMR) represents the energy expended at rest to maintain essential bodily functions, such as breathing, circulation, and cell repair.

2. Factors Influencing Metabolism: Several factors influence metabolism, including age, gender, body composition, genetics, hormone levels, diet, exercise habits, and overall health status.

Temporary Boosts vs. Permanent Changes:

1. Temporary Effects: Certain interventions, such as consuming spicy foods, caffeine, or engaging in high-intensity exercise, can temporarily increase metabolism through mechanisms such as thermogenesis or increased energy expenditure. However, these effects are typically short-lived and may not lead to long-term changes in metabolic rate.

2. Long-Term Changes: While it's possible to make lifestyle modifications that support overall metabolic health, such as building lean muscle mass through strength training or improving insulin sensitivity through dietary changes, these changes are not necessarily permanent and require ongoing maintenance.

Factors Influencing Metabolic Rate:

1. Muscle Mass: Lean muscle mass has a higher metabolic rate compared to fat tissue, meaning that individuals with a higher proportion of muscle tend to have a higher BMR. Therefore, strength training and resistance exercise can help increase muscle mass and support a higher metabolic rate over time.

2. Physical Activity: Regular physical activity, including both aerobic exercise and strength training, can temporarily increase metabolism during and after exercise sessions. Incorporating physical activity into daily routines can support overall metabolic health and energy expenditure.

3. Dietary Factors: Certain dietary factors, such as consuming adequate protein, fiber, and healthy fats, can support metabolic health and satiety. Additionally, avoiding excessive calorie restriction or yo-yo dieting, which can lower

metabolic rate and lead to metabolic adaptation, is important for maintaining a healthy metabolism.

4. Hormonal Balance: Hormones such as thyroid hormones, cortisol, insulin, and leptin play key roles in regulating metabolism. Maintaining hormonal balance through healthy lifestyle habits, adequate sleep, and stress management can support overall metabolic health.

Strategies for Supporting Metabolism:

1. Balanced Diet: Focus on consuming a balanced diet that includes a variety of nutrient-dense foods, such as lean proteins, fruits, vegetables, whole grains, and healthy fats. Avoiding excessive processed foods, sugary snacks, and refined carbohydrates can support metabolic health.

2. Regular Exercise: Incorporate regular physical activity into your routine, including both aerobic exercise and strength training. Aim for a combination of cardiovascular exercise to burn calories and strength training to build muscle mass and support a higher metabolic rate.

3. Adequate Sleep: Prioritize quality sleep, as inadequate sleep can disrupt hormone levels, appetite regulation, and metabolic function. Aim for 7-9 hours of uninterrupted sleep per night to support overall health and well-being.

4. Stress Management: Practice stress-reducing techniques such as mindfulness, meditation, deep breathing exercises, or yoga to manage stress levels and support hormonal balance.

Conclusion:

While it's possible to make lifestyle changes that support overall metabolic health and energy expenditure, the idea of permanently boosting metabolism is more complex. Rather than seeking quick fixes or magic solutions, focus on adopting sustainable lifestyle habits that support overall health and well-being. By prioritizing regular physical activity, balanced nutrition, adequate sleep, and stress management, you can optimize your metabolic health and support long-term vitality. Remember that individual factors such as genetics, age, and hormonal balance also play significant roles in metabolic regulation, so it's essential to approach metabolism holistically and with realistic expectations.

Chapter 10:

Conclusion: Embracing a Healthy Lifestyle with Fat-Burning Foods

Embracing a healthy lifestyle that incorporates fat-burning foods is a holistic approach to optimizing overall health, supporting weight management, and promoting sustainable well-being. By understanding the principles of metabolism, the role of nutrition, and the importance of lifestyle factors, individuals can make informed choices to enhance their health and vitality. Here's an extensive and comprehensive conclusion on embracing a healthy lifestyle with fat-burning foods:

Understanding Metabolism and Nutrition:

1. Metabolism: Metabolism encompasses the complex processes by which the body converts food into energy to sustain life. Basal metabolic

rate (BMR) represents the energy expended at rest, while factors such as physical activity, dietary choices, and lifestyle habits influence overall energy expenditure.

2. Nutrition: The quality of nutrition plays a crucial role in supporting metabolic health. Incorporating nutrient-dense foods such as lean proteins, fruits, vegetables, whole grains, and healthy fats provides essential nutrients while promoting satiety and metabolic function.

Importance of Fat-Burning Foods:

1. Role in Metabolism: Certain foods, such as lean proteins, high-fiber foods, spices and herbs, healthy fats, and metabolism-boosting nutrients, can support metabolic health and energy expenditure. These foods may enhance thermogenesis, promote satiety, stabilize blood sugar levels, and support muscle maintenance and growth.

2. Nutrient Density: Fat-burning foods are often nutrient-dense, providing essential vitamins, minerals, antioxidants, and phytonutrients that support overall health and well-being. By prioritizing these foods, individuals can optimize their nutritional intake and support metabolic function.

Embracing a Healthy Lifestyle:

1. Balanced Diet: Focus on consuming a balanced diet that includes a variety of fat-burning foods, along with adequate hydration and portion control. Avoiding excessive processed foods, sugary snacks, and refined carbohydrates can support metabolic health and weight management.

2. Regular Physical Activity: Incorporate regular exercise into your routine, including both aerobic exercise and strength training.

Aim for a combination of cardiovascular exercise to burn calories and strength training to build muscle mass and support a higher metabolic rate.

3. Quality Sleep: Prioritize quality sleep to support overall health and metabolic function. Aim for 7-9 hours of uninterrupted sleep per night to promote hormone balance, appetite regulation, and energy levels.

4. Stress Management: Practice stress-reducing techniques such as mindfulness, meditation, deep breathing exercises, or yoga to manage stress levels and support hormonal balance. Chronic stress can disrupt metabolism and contribute to weight gain and metabolic dysfunction.

Sustainable Habits for Long-Term Success:

1. Consistency: Embrace sustainable lifestyle habits that can be maintained long-term rather than seeking quick fixes or fad diets. Consistency is key for seeing lasting results and maintaining metabolic health over time.

2. Flexibility: Allow for flexibility in your diet and exercise routine, recognizing that balance and moderation are essential for overall well-being. Avoid rigid rules or restrictions that may lead to feelings of deprivation or burnout.

3. Mindful Eating: Practice mindful eating by paying attention to hunger cues, eating slowly, and savoring the flavors and textures of food. Avoid emotional eating or eating out of boredom, and focus on nourishing your body with nutrient-rich foods.

Conclusion:

Embracing a healthy lifestyle with fat-burning foods is not just about achieving short-term weight loss goals but about supporting overall health, vitality, and well-being. By prioritizing nutrient-dense foods, regular physical activity, quality sleep, and stress management techniques, individuals can optimize their metabolic health and enjoy the benefits of sustained energy, improved mood, and enhanced vitality. Remember that embracing a healthy lifestyle is a journey, and small, consistent changes can lead to significant and lasting results over time. With dedication, mindfulness, and a focus on holistic well-being, anyone can achieve their health and wellness goals and thrive in the long term.

Recap of Key Points

Recapping key points is essential for reinforcing the main concepts discussed and providing a concise summary of the extensive information covered. Here's an extensive and comprehensive recap of the key points highlighted throughout the discussion on embracing a healthy lifestyle with fat-burning foods:

Understanding Metabolism and Nutrition:

1. Metabolism: Metabolism is the body's process of converting food into energy to sustain life. Basal metabolic rate (BMR) represents energy expenditure at rest, while factors like physical activity, diet, and lifestyle influence overall energy balance.

2. Nutrition: Prioritize nutrient-dense foods such as lean proteins, fruits, vegetables, whole grains, and healthy fats. These foods provide essential nutrients, promote satiety, and support metabolic function.

Importance of Fat-Burning Foods:

1. Role in Metabolism: Fat-burning foods can enhance thermogenesis, promote satiety, stabilize blood sugar levels, and support muscle maintenance and growth, ultimately aiding in weight management and metabolic health.

2. Nutrient Density: Fat-burning foods are often rich in essential vitamins, minerals, antioxidants, and phytonutrients, which support overall health and well-being.

Embracing a Healthy Lifestyle:

1. Balanced Diet: Consume a balanced diet that includes a variety of fat-burning foods, while avoiding processed foods, sugary snacks, and refined carbohydrates.

2. Regular Physical Activity: Incorporate both aerobic exercise and strength training into your routine to burn calories, build muscle, and support a higher metabolic rate.

3. Quality Sleep: Prioritize adequate sleep to promote hormone balance, appetite regulation, and metabolic function.

4. Stress Management: Practice stress-reducing techniques such as mindfulness, meditation, or yoga to support hormonal balance and metabolic health.

Sustainable Habits for Long-Term Success:

1. Consistency: Adopt sustainable lifestyle habits that can be maintained long-term, emphasizing consistency over quick fixes or fad diets.

2. Flexibility: Allow for flexibility in your diet and exercise routine, avoiding rigid rules or restrictions that may lead to deprivation or burnout.

3. Mindful Eating: Pay attention to hunger cues, eat slowly, and focus on nourishing your body with nutrient-rich foods to support overall well-being.

Conclusion:

Embracing a healthy lifestyle with fat-burning foods involves prioritizing nutrient-dense foods, regular physical activity, quality sleep, and stress management techniques. By consistently implementing these habits, individuals can optimize their metabolic health, support weight management, and enjoy sustained energy and vitality. Remember that small, consistent changes can lead to significant and lasting results over time, ultimately promoting overall health and well-being.

Encouragement for Sustainable Changes

Encouragement for sustainable changes is crucial for individuals embarking on a journey towards a healthier lifestyle with fat-burning foods. Making lasting changes requires dedication, patience, and resilience, and providing support and motivation can help individuals stay committed to their goals. Here's an extensive and comprehensive exploration of strategies for encouraging sustainable changes:

Understanding the Journey:

1. Acknowledge Progress: Celebrate every step of the journey, no matter how small. Recognize and celebrate achievements, milestones, and improvements, whether they're related to diet, exercise, or overall well-being.

2. Embrace Setbacks: Understand that setbacks are a natural part of the process. Instead of viewing them as failures, see them as opportunities for learning and growth. Encourage resilience and perseverance in the face of challenges.

Providing Support:

1. Build a Support System: Surround yourself with a supportive network of friends, family members, or health professionals who can offer encouragement, accountability, and guidance along the way. Share your goals and progress with others to stay motivated and accountable.

2. Accountability Partners: Find an accountability partner or join a community or group with similar health and wellness goals. Having someone to share your journey with can provide motivation, encouragement, and accountability.

Cultivating Positive Mindset:

1. Focus on Non-Scale Victories: Shift the focus away from solely weight-related goals and instead celebrate non-scale victories such as increased energy levels, improved mood, better sleep, and enhanced overall well-being.

2. Practice Self-Compassion: Be kind to yourself and practice self-compassion, especially during challenging times. Avoid self-criticism or negative self-talk and instead focus on positive affirmations and self-care practices.

Setting Realistic Expectations:

1. Focus on Long-Term Health: Emphasize the importance of long-term health and well-being over quick fixes or short-term results. Encourage sustainable lifestyle changes that prioritize health, vitality, and overall well-being.

2. Break Goals into Manageable Steps: Help individuals break down their goals into smaller, achievable steps. Set realistic expectations and encourage progress over perfection.

Celebrating Success:

1. Acknowledge Achievements: Celebrate achievements, no matter how small. Acknowledge and reward progress to reinforce positive behaviors and motivate continued effort.

2. Reflect on Progress: Take time to reflect on progress and accomplishments regularly. Keep a journal or record milestones to track how far you've come and remind yourself of the progress made.

Providing Encouragement:

1. Offer Words of Affirmation: Offer words of encouragement, support, and affirmation to individuals as they navigate their health and wellness journey. Provide positive feedback and praise for their efforts and accomplishments.

2. Lead by Example: Be a role model by demonstrating healthy habits and behaviors in your own life. Share your own experiences, successes, and challenges to inspire and motivate others on their journey.

Conclusion:

Encouraging sustainable changes involves providing support, cultivating a positive mindset, setting realistic expectations, celebrating success, and offering words of encouragement. By fostering a supportive environment and empowering individuals to embrace their health and wellness journey, we can inspire lasting change and promote overall well-being. Remember that every step forward, no matter how small, brings individuals closer to their goals and contributes to a healthier, happier life.

Commitment to Long-Term Health and Wellness

Commitment to long-term health and wellness is a journey that involves making sustainable lifestyle changes, prioritizing self-care, and fostering a positive relationship with one's health. It requires dedication, perseverance, and a proactive approach to maintaining overall well-being. Here's an extensive and comprehensive exploration of the importance of commitment to long-term health and wellness:

Understanding Long-Term Health and Wellness:

1. Holistic Approach: Long-term health and wellness encompass physical, mental, emotional, and spiritual well-being. It involves nurturing every aspect of one's health to achieve a balanced and fulfilling life.

2. Preventive Care: Prioritizing long-term health involves taking proactive measures to prevent illness and disease before they occur. This includes regular health screenings, vaccinations, and lifestyle modifications to reduce risk factors.

Benefits of Long-Term Health and Wellness:

1. Improved Quality of Life: Investing in long-term health and wellness can lead to a higher quality of life, characterized by greater energy, vitality, and resilience to stressors.

2. Reduced Risk of Chronic Disease* Adopting healthy lifestyle habits can lower the risk of developing chronic diseases such as heart disease, diabetes, obesity, and certain cancers, promoting longevity and well-being.

3. Enhanced Mental Health: Prioritizing mental health through practices such as stress management, mindfulness, and therapy can lead to reduced anxiety, depression, and overall improved emotional well-being.

Commitment to Sustainable Lifestyle Changes:

1. Consistent Habits: Long-term health and wellness require consistent habits and behaviors that support overall well-being. This includes maintaining a balanced diet, engaging in regular physical activity, getting adequate sleep, and managing stress effectively.

2. Mindful Eating: Adopting mindful eating practices, such as listening to hunger and fullness cues, savoring food, and choosing nutrient-dense options, promotes a healthy relationship with food and supports long-term dietary habits.

Strategies for Long-Term Success:

1. Goal Setting: Set specific, measurable, achievable, relevant, and time-bound (SMART) goals that align with long-term health and

wellness objectives. Break goals down into manageable steps and track progress over time.

2. Self-Reflection: Regularly reflect on personal values, priorities, and motivations related to health and wellness. Identify areas for improvement and reassess goals to ensure they remain relevant and meaningful.

3. Seeking Support: Build a supportive network of friends, family members, healthcare professionals, or wellness coaches who can provide encouragement, accountability, and guidance on the journey to long-term health and wellness.

4. Adaptability: Remain flexible and adaptable in the face of challenges or setbacks. Recognize that progress may not always be linear and be willing to adjust goals or strategies as needed to stay on track.

Cultivating Resilience:

1. Positive Mindset: Cultivate a positive mindset by focusing on strengths, resilience, and growth opportunities. Practice gratitude, optimism, and self-compassion to navigate challenges and setbacks with resilience and grace.

2. Learning from Setbacks: View setbacks as opportunities for learning and growth rather than failures. Identify lessons learned, adjust strategies as needed, and use setbacks as motivation to continue moving forward on the journey to long-term health and wellness.

Conclusion:

Commitment to long-term health and wellness is a lifelong journey that involves making sustainable lifestyle changes, prioritizing self-care, and fostering resilience. By adopting consistent habits, setting meaningful goals, seeking support, and cultivating a positive mindset, individuals can empower themselves to live healthier, happier, and more fulfilling lives. Remember that the journey to long-term health and wellness is unique to each individual and requires patience, dedication, and a steadfast commitment to personal well-being.